Contents

List of Tables   xi
Foreword   xiii
     Thomas N. Wise, M.D.

1 Introduction and Overview of the Historical Basis of Consultation-Liaison Psychiatry   1

The Importance of a Consultation-Liaison
   Psychiatry Manual   1
Overview of the Manual   5
Historical Perspective on Psychiatric
   Consultation   10
      Historical Overview of Consultation-Liaison
         Clinical Practice   12
      Historical Developments in Scientific Theories
         of Psychobiology   13
References   15
Appendix: Conceptual History of Psychosomatic
   Medicine   20

2 Setting the Stage   23

Consulting in a New Setting   23
Meeting the Staff   24
      Administrators   25
      Secretaries/Clerks   25
      Social Workers   26
      Psychologists and Other Mental Health
         Professionals   28
      Nursing Staff   30
      Other Specialized Service Staff   31
      Members of the Clergy   32
      House Staff   33
Establishing the Consultant-Consultee
   Relationship   33

Attitude of the Primary Physician Toward
   Psychiatry   34
Attitude of the Psychiatric Consultant Toward
   the Consultee   34
Consultee Practice Patterns As They Relate to
   Consultation   35
Becoming Familiar With the Consultee
   Specialty   36
Becoming Familiar With the Institution   37
Teaching   37
Working With a Known Service   38
Role of the Psychiatrist as Consultant   39
References   40

3 **Initiating the Consultation**   **41**

Prearrangements   42
The Consultation Information Card   42
The Consultee   44
Calling Mechanisms   45
   Call Coverage   46
      Paging Systems   46
      Triage   47
Information to Request   49
   Rationale   49
   Specific Pieces of Information   50
Recording and Conveying the Information   51
Conclusions   52
References   52

4 **Contacting the Referring Service**   **55**

Timing   56
Whom to Contact   57
Information Sought   58
   Nature of the Clinical Problem   58
      "Medical" Aspects   58
      "Psychiatric" Aspects   61

Manual of Psychiatric Consultation

Nada L. Stotland, M.D.

*Associate Professor of Clinical Psychiatry
and Obstetrics and Gynecology
and
Director of Psychiatric Education
Department of Psychiatry
University of Chicago
Chicago, Illinois*

Thomas R. Garrick, M.D.

*Chief of Psychiatry
Wadsworth Division
West Los Angeles Veterans Administration
Medical Center
and
Associate Professor of Psychiatry
Department of Psychiatry
University of California, Los Angeles
Los Angeles, California*

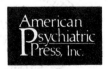

American
Psychiatric
Press, Inc.

Washington, DC
London, England

NOTE: The authors have worked to ensure that all information in this book concerning drug dosages, schedules, and routes of administration is accurate as of the time of publication and consistent with standards set by the U.S. Food and Drug Administration and the general medical community. As medical research and practice advance, however, therapeutic standards may change. For this reason and because human and mechanical errors sometimes occur, we recommend that readers follow the advice of a physician who is directly involved in their care or the care of a member of their family.

Copyright © 1990 American Psychiatric Press, Inc.
ALL RIGHTS RESERVED
Manufactured in the United States of America
First Edition

93 92 91 90 4 3 2 1

The paper used in this publication meets the minimum requirements of the American National Standard for Information Sciences – Permanence of Paper for Printed Library Materials, ANSI Z39.48–1984.

Library of Congress Cataloging-in-Publication Data

Stotland, Nada Logan.
  Manual of psychiatric consultation / Nada L. Stotland, Thomas R. Garrick.
      p.   cm.
  Includes bibliographical references.
  ISBN 0-88048-311-3
  1. Consultation-liaison psychiatry. I. Garrick, Thomas R., 1950-
  II. Title.
  [DNLM: 1. Hospitals, General. 2. Referral and Consultation. 3. Psychiatry. WM 64 S888m]
  RC455.2.C65S76   1990
  616.89'0068—dc20
  DNLM/DLC
  for Library of Congress   89-18511
                                                                        CIP

British Cataloguing in Publication Data

A CIP record is available from the British Library

The Precipitant for Calling the
    Consultation   63
Urgency   64
Location and Availability of Patient   65
Determining Who Is the Psychiatrist
    Responsible for a Given Consultation   66
Making a Contract for the Initial Consultation   67
Informing the Patient   67
Time, Duration, and Content of Initial
    Consultation   69
References   70

5 The First Visit to the Hospital Unit   71

Finding Out Who Is Taking Care of the Patient   72
Staff Relationships   76
The Patient's Chart   78
When to Review the Chart   78
Overview   79
    The "Old Chart"   79
    The "Face Sheet"   79
    Admission Notes   80
    Progress Notes   80
    Nursing and Other Staff Notes   81
    Vital Signs   81
    Laboratory Values and Other Test
      Results   82
    Other Consultations   82
Visitors   83
Conclusions   85
References   85

6 Seeing the Patient   87

Unique Issues in Psychiatric Consultation   88
Patient Consent and Preparation   88
Confidentiality   89
The Contract—Conflicts   92

Conduct of the Interview   93
    Technical Questions   93
    Explaining the Consultant's Presence:
      Relieving Anxiety and Soliciting
      Cooperation   95
    The Patient Who Refuses Psychiatric
      Interview   97
    Interview Content   98
    Mental Status Examination   100
Physical Examination   102
Observing the Environment   103
Conveying Preliminary Impressions to the
    Patient   104
References   106

7 What to Do Before Leaving the Medical Unit

109

Another Look at the Available Information   110
    The Chart   110
    The Staff   110
    Family and Friends   112
The Need for Outside Information   114
    Past Medical Records   114
    Other Sources   114
Administrative and Legal Issues   116
Urgent Recommendations   118
Sharing First Impressions   122
References   124

8 Writing Up the Consultation

127

Written Psychiatric Consultation Document   128
    Title   128
    Date, Time, and Sources of Information   129
    Identifying Statement   129
    History   132
    Mental Status Examination   133
    Formulations   135

Recommendations   137
    Further Workup   137
    Consultee Management   137
    Consultant Management   139
The Limited, Noncomprehensive
   Consultation   140
Legal Implications   140
Conclusions   140
References   141
Appendix A: Suggested Outline for the Written
   Psychiatric Consultation   143
Appendix B: An Example of a Computer-Assisted
   Data Base as a Supplement to the Written
   Consultation   144

9 Recommendations   **149**

Liaison   149
Types of Recommendations   152
   Further Diagnostic Workup   152
    Psychiatric Workup   152
    Consultations: Neuropsychological and
      Psychological Testing   153
    Consultations: Medical and
      Neurological   153
    Medical Workup: Laboratory Tests   154
    Medical Workup: Differential
      Diagnosis   154
    Consultations: Nonmedical   155
   Behavior Management   156
    Provisions for Patient Safety   156
    Restraints   157
    Monitoring of Visitors   159
    Discharge Against Medical Advice   160
    Consent to Treatment   161
    Discharge and Dangerousness   162
   Treatment   164
    Social Intervention   164
    Psychotherapeutic Treatment   167

Psychopharmacological Treatment   167
Special Referral   169
Transfer and Referral   169
Psychiatric Follow-up: Delineation of
    Responsibility   170
References   171
Appendix: Sample Briefing Sheet for Nursing
    Assistants Assigned to Monitor Suicidal
    Patients   173

**10 Follow-Through, Follow-Up, and Closing
the Consultation**   **177**

Assessing the Need for Follow-up   177
Goals for Follow-up   182
Implementation   185
Discharge Planning   188
Ending the Consultation   190
References   191

**11 Role of the Consultation-Liaison
Psychiatrist as a Medical Educator**   **193**

Training of Nonpsychiatric Physicians   193
Training Psychiatric Residents in
    Consultation-Liaison   196
Training of Medical Students in
    Consultation-Liaison Psychiatry   202
References   203

**12 Consultation-Liaison in a Changing
World of Psychiatry**   **205**

The Benefits of Consultation-Liaison Psychiatry to
    the Medical Unit   206
    Diagnosis   206
    Treatment   207
    Funding of Modern Medicine and
        Consultation-Liaison Psychiatry:
        Cost-Effectiveness   208

Cost Savings Resulting From Psychiatric
    Consultation   210
Stress on Inpatient Wards and the Psychiatric
    Consultant   212
Medicolegal Issues   213
    Danger to Self   213
    Danger to Others   215
    Informed Consent for Medical
        Procedures   215
    Psychotropic Medication Side Effects   217
    Electroconvulsive Therapy   218
    Confidentiality   218
Service Standards   219
Conclusions   223
References   223

Index   227

List of Tables

Table 11-1. Knowledge objectives for residents in consultation-liaison psychiatry   198

Table 11-2. Skills objectives for residents in consultation-liaison psychiatry   200

Table 12-1. Quality assurance outline for medical-care personnel   221

Foreword

The psychiatric consultation in a general medical setting is the most public clinical task that a psychiatrist performs. The psychiatrist will be observed by a variety of individuals. This public role compounds the difficulties of consultation work, which include inconvenient scheduling, the specter of dire illnesses, and the direct encounter with pain and disfigurement.

The great satisfaction of being a consultation psychiatrist is, however, to work with a variety of fascinating clinical problems in a medical culture that affirms psychiatry's medical heritage. The consultation psychiatrist becomes the ambassador of psychiatry to our medical colleagues. Although there is increasing pressure upon psychiatry to share its clinical arena with other mental health providers, only the psychiatrist can fully integrate the various perspectives from which each patient must be viewed.

P. R. McHugh and P. R. Slavney (*The Perspectives of Psychiatry.* Baltimore, MD, Johns Hopkins University Press, 1983) have elegantly described the variety of methods that are utilized in clinical psychiatry. Nowhere is this variety of methods better demonstrated than in consultation psychiatry. The consultation psychiatrist must be able to view his or her patients from a biologic perspective that utilizes a medical model. The medical model considers signs and symptoms that may ultimately correlate with a clear pathophysiologic disorder. The psychiatrist must also utilize the life history methodology whereby each patient is a unique human being who subjectively experiences a variety of environmental and personal stresses. This is the perspective in which psychodynamic psychiatry resides. In addition, the consultation psychiatrist sees a variety of motivated behaviors through which the goal of reduction in tension is achieved. Addictive disorders and eating disorders may best be investigated within such a frame of reference. Finally, the realm of personality as expressed through trait differences is a final methodology that complements the preceding three approaches. Intersubject personality differences, such as the ability of the patient to be more or less extroverted, emotionally stable, or agreeable, must be appreciated and understood in the context of the patient's ability to cope with the stress of illness and treatment. Only the psychiatric physician can integrate all such perspectives.

Thus when asked to see a patient who complains of disabling anxiety and is demanding attention and medication from the nursing staff, the psychiatrist must consider a variety of options. What is the patient's medical status? Is an endocrine disorder augmenting his or her anxiety? How have the patient's prior life experiences affected the present situation in the hospital? Is the patient a substance abuser? Finally, what is his or her basic personality type? Such data are often difficult to obtain, and immediate answers are not always forthcoming. Nevertheless, by ongoing interaction with the patient and the medical staff, and by considering other sources of information, the psychiatrist can begin to fully understand the patient's predicament both in terms of individual diagnostic categorization directed toward the patient, and in terms of a small–systems context that helps explain reactions among the treating staff.

Is consultation-liaison psychiatry a subspecialty? (See Houpt JL: The future of consultation-liaison psychiatry as a psychiatric subspecialty, in *The Future of Psychiatry as a Medical Specialty.* Edited by Yager J. Washington, DC, American Psychiatric Press, 1989, pp 47–56.) Because the focus of care includes all age ranges, the arena of practice seems to define consultation work. This work is done in both ambulatory and institutional medical settings. All psychiatrists should have basic skills in performing a consultation, but clearly some psychiatrists have and will continue to take advanced training in this area. Sophisticated techniques of managing the chronic pain patient and the oncology patient, or ongoing work with a primary care program, underscore the variety of consultation work.

Whether consultation-liaison psychiatry is indeed sufficiently unique from general psychiatry to be considered for formal subspecialty status remains to be seen. However, the *Manual of Psy-*

chiatric Consultation demonstrates the complexity and depth of the clinical interaction with such patients and with attending health-care providers. This important volume provides both the content and the process necessary to perform the consultation. Drs. Stotland and Garrick, skilled educators, within consultation psychiatry, exemplify the clinical wisdom that is needed by a subspecialist. The body of knowledge within this book suggests that consultation psychiatry is indeed a subspecialty that should be familiar to all psychiatrists as well as a focused career pattern for some.

Thomas N. Wise, M.D.

1

Introduction and Overview of the Historical Basis of Consultation-Liaison Psychiatry

This manual offers practicing psychiatrists, teachers, and trainees an in-depth, orderly analysis of and guide to the process of consultation psychiatry in the general hospital. For the psychiatrist either established or working in an existing academic or private consultation service, we provide a structure and working approach to the consultation-liaison process. Finally, throughout the manual, we address issues critical to today's consultation-liaison psychiatrist, including medicolegal formulations of practice, rapidly evolving ethical issues in medicine in general and in psychiatry in particular, cost-effectiveness, risk management, and the impact of new health-care delivery constraints.

THE IMPORTANCE OF A CONSULTATION-LIAISON PSYCHIATRY MANUAL

World-wide, more and more psychiatrists are practicing on medical and surgical wards of hospitals in order to address the psychiatric needs of medically hospitalized patients (Freyberger et al. 1985; Iwasaka 1979). However, as these psychiatrists have discovered, this new clinical setting requires approaches to diagnosis and treatment that differ from those used in other clinical situations. In such a setting, the consultation-liaison psychiatrist commonly encounters a wide array of medical and psychiatric problems that the office- or inpatient-based psychiatrist rarely sees. These medicopsychiatric clinical problems include malingering, conversion, drug withdrawal, and reactions to medical illness. Several useful texts (Hackett 1987; Kimball 1979; Pasnau 1975; Strain and Grossman 1975) address the specific clinical issues commonly encountered by consultation-liaison psychiatrists; however, few actually analyze the process necessary to working in this setting. These texts ignore, for example, the degree to which consultation-liaison psychiatry demands and provides opportunities for unique interventions. By contrast, this volume will provide a comprehensive, current, and reasoned guide to consulting in this clinical setting.

Thus, for example, the consultation-liaison psychiatrist must understand how the clinical environment affects how he or she establishes and maintains *therapeutic alliances*. In the general hospital, psychiatrist and patient collaborate on a different basis than they do in the outpatient or inpatient psychiatric practice. In outpatient or inpatient practice, the patient commonly initiates psychiatric treatment when he or she seeks out the counsel of the therapist because the patient is experiencing psychological pain (Beebe and Rosenbaum 1975). In such cases, the patient may be referred to the particular treating psychiatrist by a friend, a nonpsychiatric physician, or another psychiatrist, or may choose psychotherapeutic assistance of a general or a particular nature from a professional associated with a particular clinic. However, even when the patient is not financially able to select a therapist, he or she nevertheless has some independent role in choosing to be seen.

In marked contrast, the consultation-liaison psychiatrist generally participates in the patient's case at the request of a nonpsychiatric physician. That is, the patient does not directly choose to be diagnosed or treated by the consultation-liaison practitioner. A nonpsychiatric physician, who may only superficially know the patient, arranges for a psychiatrist, who is unknown to the patient (and possibly to the physician as well), to assess and address the patient's emotional and cognitive status. Usually, a hospitalized patient does not even have time to consult with family, friends, or other members of his or her support system before agreeing to be examined. Not surprisingly, the patient's sense of helplessness is compounded by the psychological and behavioral difficulties that triggered the consult originally: suspicion, anger, hurt, fright, and narcissistic injury. If the primary physician arranges the referrals awkwardly, he or she may further contribute to the patient's discomfort. As a result of all these factors, patients may respond with varying degrees of intensity to the consult or to the consultation-liaison psychiatrist. Under these circumstances, the consultation-liaison psychiatrist must carefully ascertain the patient's mental status and level of social functioning while quickly establishing a measure of trust in a confused, angry, and/or suspicious patient. For both the patient and the consultation-liaison psychiatrist, the success of this process determines whether or not the therapeutic alliance will succeed.

Unlike other psychiatric settings, the consultation-liaison situation provides an opportunity for a wide range of distinctive *therapeutic interventions*. Confronting challenges to his or her biological, as well as psychological, integrity, the consultation-liaison patient is often already in crisis by the time the consultant is called in. The hospitalization has usually distanced the patient from his or her usual sources of social and emotional support. Thus, the patient's medical illness may intensify previous personal problems. Alternatively, the hospitalization may distance the patient from such problems; this new perspective renders his or her problems more manageable. Finally, the patient may displace personal problems, such as hopelessness with one's achievements, onto the medical situation, intensifying the degree of discouragement and disability and making the diagnosis even more difficult.

Consultation-liaison practice also contrasts markedly with practice in the outpatient setting. In the consultation-liaison setting, the primary referring physician and the consultation-liaison psychiatrist have already begun to decide the appropriate method(s) of treatment and have identified the goals of the interventions. Before the patient has even been interviewed, such prior agreements raise the question of whether the patient actually has or can have a significant role in deciding the initial direction of any treatment, or has or can have an accurate preconception about any caregiver. Typically, in fact, the patient experiences outpatient treatment as more self-directed than in the medical hospital, where he or she is not even seen unless the attending physician requests the consultation from the consultation-liaison psychiatrist.

But, the consultation-liaison clinical setting also affects the psychiatrist's professional role because it confronts him or her with complicated alliances. Called in by the medical team, the psychiatrist may have trouble determining to whom he or she owes a primary allegiance (Lipowski 1975). The psychiatric consultant may find that responsibility to the patient conflicts with the needs of the service requesting psychiatric consultation for behavioral control. For example, the consultant may be caught between a busy medical service that wants a passive and compliant patient and a patient who is dissatisfied with the service received. More problematic, the psychiatrist may encounter situations in which psychiatric goals conflict with short-term medical management aims. For example, a medical team might maintain a drug abuser on high doses of narcotics to facilitate current adjustment in the medical system.

Such circumstances are far from optimal for the consultant who must initiate a psychotherapeutic relationship. Indeed, to the unexperienced, the possibilities for failure appear insurmountable. However, by addressing these considerations directly we hope to provide a framework that minimizes the potential negative consequences of such complicated arrangements and thus increases the consultation-liaison psychiatrist's ability to assist the service, the medical team, and the patient.

Because the most successful consultations occur in the milieu of an ongoing "liaison" relationship between the psychiatric consultant and the various members of the medical and paramedical team, the consultation-liaison psychiatrist must consider each aspect of the milieu when he or she evaluates the patient's problem (Lipowski 1975). In order to obtain information, the psychiatric consultant must deal with a wide and changing array of other medical and paramedical specialists, administrative personnel, and legal personnel. While another physician has primary medical responsibility, the consultant must still make decisions that significantly affect the care obtained by the patient. Constrained by time, the consultant must all too often make clinical decisions without adequate information. Taken together, these demands and constraints suggest that the consultant's ability to make the best clinical decisions depends directly on how well he or she understands the hospital-patient system.

While the emphasis of this manual is on consultation and liaison psychiatry as practiced in the inpatient setting, the principles discussed are applicable to the outpatient setting as well. Currently there is a dearth of information about the variations in structure and interest in the use of outpatient consultation-liaison activities (Fava et al. 1987; Wolcott et al. 1984). With the current shift in hospital utilization from inpatient activities to ambulatory care, "psychosomatic" clinics will become increasingly prominent. These clinics also may serve a population that is not effectively served by more traditional outpatient psychiatric and medical services (Fava et al. 1987; Schwartz et al. 1987). From a didactic perspective, however, we believe the intensity of the inpatient consultation-liaison experience provides the best model for exploring the process of this form of psychiatric intervention.

In the rest of this manual we will focus on how the consultant should understand the constraints and demands of the settings in order to provide the best care for medically hospitalized patients who need psychiatric treatment.

OVERVIEW OF THE MANUAL

In pursuit of this end, we provide a step-by-step analysis of the process of consultation. To make the process understandable to the reader, we will present the rationale for each step in the process and then discuss detailed practical guidelines for how to accomplish each step in the consultation. We will use clinical materials liberally to illustrate the consultation process and attend both to typical problems encountered in daily practice and to typical solutions to those problems. For ease and clarity, we have organized the manual in rough chronological order, working from initial involvement to recommendations to new developments in the field.

In the remaining section of Chapter 1, we briefly outline the history of consultation-liaison psychiatry. In recent years, neurobiological research has profoundly affected the treatment of patients with so-called "psychosomatic illnesses" by linking psychological processes of emotion, behavior, and brain function to the pathophysiology and anatomic pathology of the other organ systems. Similarly, our understanding of brain-body irregularity has been transformed as we have discovered the neurotransmitters that operate in particular areas of the brain to modulate the function of individual organs. These scientific developments parallel the increase in the number of psychiatrists who have become integral members of the team of clinical medical specialists (Schwab 1989). In response to these changes in clinical practice, segments of medical school and residency training have been allocated to the subject area of consultation-liaison, keeping pace with the increased involvement of psychiatrists in medical decision making.

In Chapter 2, we detail the early phases of the psychiatrist's involvement on the medical ward, with particular emphasis on new settings. Optimal practice depends on the psychiatrist establishing a comfortable relationship with the medical team and becoming an accessible and contributing member. The psychiatrist must define his or her unique contribution to the medical workup, treatment, and discharge plan. In Chapter 2, we will present various methods for approaching these tasks with each type of staff.

The mechanism of consultation intake is examined in Chapter 3. Consultations may represent a perceived or actual emergency, a confusing diagnostic dilemma, or a situation requiring psychiatric involvement for medicolegal reasons. In every case, if the medical or surgical ward is to function smoothly, the psychiatrist must be able to provide timely assistance whenever needed. We outline the optimal methods to channel consultations to the consultation service in order to avoid confusing or irritating the consultee service. The consultant should always strive to communicate clearly with the service and staff to facilitate the volume of consultation requests and ensure that he or she is consistently available.

In Chapter 4, we discuss various factors to be considered when contacting the primary physician who requested a psychiatric consultation. Because its goal is to establish the contract between the two physicians, the initial communication between the consultee physician and the consultation-liaison psychiatrist is a most critical phase in the consultation. Thus, the consultation-liaison psychiatrist must consider when to approach the staff, how to identify the physician to contact when there are several members of a treatment team, and how to determine who can provide the most useful information to the consultant. As outlined in this chapter, the psychiatrist's goals are to understand how the service views the problems for which it is seeking help, to obtain information essential to the psychiatric workup, and to establish the psychiatrist as a physician with both a medical and a psychosocial view of the illness process. We then suggest ways to structure early interactions with the medical team in order to develop a successful contract for a working relationship.

Next, in Chapter 5, we examine the psychiatric consultant's first visit to the hospital floor. As many a patient and family know, information gathering can be a difficult process in the medical hospital. We suggest methods for gathering psychosocial and medical information by contacting each of the important staff members, family, and visitors who interact with and know the patient best. We detail a range of ways to gather information, because each perspective provides valuable data about how the patient functions in different situations under different demands and can make the consultation easier.

We then, in Chapter 6, delineate the consultation-liaison patient interview and how it differs from the patient interview conducted on an inpatient psychiatric ward or in an outpatient setting. As we suggested earlier, for example, the environment itself may be the focus of or contribute greatly to the patient's psychological distress. In addition, the psychiatrist may need to perform a limited physical examination such as a neurological evaluation in order to develop a differential diagnosis. In Chapter 6, other issues, such as confidentiality, are addressed that further differentiate the hospital from other diagnostic sites. Finally, the chapter touches on methods for dealing with the uncooperative patient and managing conflicts among staff members.

Initially, many psychiatrists are uncomfortable practicing on a medical ward for a variety of reasons. The psychiatric consultant copes with that discomfort when he or she is comfortable with the environmental complexities and the medical uncertainties. Our manual focuses on teaching the consultant to recognize these complexities and uncertainties as the first stage in learning to manage them.

Reflecting our concern with the consultation process, we next (Chapter 7) review what the psychiatric consultant must do after interviewing the patient for the first time and before leaving the ward. What steps should the consultant take, for example, if the evaluation reveals a dangerous psychiatric condition requiring immediate attention or a deteriorating medical condition mistakenly attributed to psychological stress? More commonly, the patient interview, the initial discussions with the staff, and/or the observation of the environment leave the consultant with several tentative but incomplete impressions of the case. In order to flush out those impressions, the consultant may take steps to expeditiously obtain information (such as the old chart, pathology, lab results, or police files) that would ensure more precise evaluation. We end the chapter by discussing strategies for effective intervention, including early contact with the physician, the nurses, or the support staff.

Having taken the reader through a complete consultation, we next explain how to write a psychiatric consultation. In Chapter 8, we examine the considerations that dictate what information is included in the written document—a key concern—because the length of the report is inversely proportional to the likelihood that it will be read. Thus, the psychiatric consultant must decide what information is most appropriate and useful for a variety of teaching, clinical, and documentary purposes. We offer both scheme and rationale for each suggestion for the written consultation. Also touched upon are the issues of confidentiality, documentation of consent, and documentation of reactions toward current and previous treatments.

The types of formal recommendations imparted in the consultation process are examined in Chapter 9. In making recommendations, the psychiatric consultant must be cognizant both of the realities of the medical or surgical service's capacities and of how much he or she plans to be involved in implementing these recommendations. In this chapter, we will present three tentative categories of recommendations. In the first category, the consultant identifies for the consultee team further psychiatric and social diagnostic workup needed, patient observations, treatment trials, drug screening, hypnosis/Amytal interviews, and psychological testing. In the second category, the consultant may recommend medical workups (such as laboratory tests and medical and radiological procedures) and initial management (such as "sitters," restraints, physical arrangements for promoting safety, warning of potential victims of violence, and discharge against medical advice). In the third category, the consultant makes recommendations about further treatment, including pharmacological treatments, brief psychodynamic psychotherapy, and relatively minimal support and social interventions (including how to arrange to place patients in nursing homes or other medical-care facilities).

After establishing the types of recommendations the psychiatric consultant can make, we address how to follow up, follow through, and close a consultation. In Chapter 10, we outline such critical components as attention to the patient and the explicitly (and sometimes implicitly) expressed needs of the consultee service. Of course, everyone's perception of an effective follow-up recaps and depends on the clarity with which the psychiatric team determined the goals of intervention in the earliest phases of the consultation process.

More generally, in Chapter 11, we focus on the role of the consultation-liaison psychiatrist as an educator in the general hospital setting. We discuss how the consultation-liaison psychiatrist can teach other nonpsychiatric physicians, nurses, and other paramedical staff to observe the cognitive and emotional status of their patients, and to identify and to attend to their patients' basic emotional needs. The consultation psychiatrist's role as educator is most intensely centered on psychiatric and nonpsychiatric residents and medical students. Mandatory for psychiatric residents, consultation-liaison training provides an ideal opportunity for the student to observe and be observed by senior staff in the process of clinical work. For medical students in particular, the consultation process allows involvement not possible in other psychiatric settings. In this medical setting, medical students learn that many psychiatric syndromes are secondary to medical illness or medications and that physiological disorder all too often masquerades as "psychological" disturbance. Further, the consultation-liaison setting ideally demonstrates normal emotional reactions to medical illness, to grief, and to the difficulties experienced when coping with loss of physical integrity.

In our final chapter, we examine new developments in the practice of consultation-liaison psychiatry. As medicine becomes increasingly subspecialized, the consultation-liaison psychiatrist is increasingly crucial to the primary-care physician's integration of psychological, social, and biological factors that contribute to a patient's disease. Currently, hospital reimbursement plans commonly recognize that the patient suffering from a psychiatric disability may need a longer period of hospitalization. The consultation-liaison psychiatrist thus becomes involved in treatment not only to facilitate efficient treatment and discharge of patients having emotional difficulties but also to appropriately identify psychiatric diagnoses essential to ensure that the hospital will be adequately reimbursed. More and more research into resource utilization demonstrates the positive effect of psychiatric intervention in cutting length of stay in the hospital (Levitan and Kornfeld 1981; Lyons et al. 1986) and in reducing the use of other high-cost medical resources (Mumford et al. 1984).

We also outline the role the consultation-liaison psychiatrist plays in risk management in the medical hospital. Many of the medicolegal issues of psychiatric hospitalization (such as civil commitment, duty to warn, duty to restrain, and informed consent) also occur in the general hospital. In the general hospital, however, different techniques are needed to address these issues because of the architecture of the wards and because the staff lacks specialized training. The consultation-liaison psychiatrist's expertise can also clarify other medicolegal problems, including informed consent, Do Not Resuscitate (DNR) orders, confidentiality, and family discord. In the final chapter, guidelines are offered on how to manage various problem situations.

As with all other medical services, consultation-liaison psychiatry requires a quality assurance plan. Therefore, we end Chapter 12 by presenting an outline for quality assurance standards including (a) educational and professional background, (b) departmental policies and procedures, (c) continuous, targeted, and incident-specific monitors, (d) employee evaluations, and (e) focused reviews.

HISTORICAL PERSPECTIVE ON PSYCHIATRIC CONSULTATION

We recognize that clinical reality and the practicalities of modern medicine often make it difficult to implement an "ideal" model of the consultation process. However, with an ideal or a set of considerations in mind, the psychiatric consultant can select those elements necessary and possible in a given clinical situation and recognize those pieces of information not obtained or those steps not performed. Before we can consider an ideal model of the consultation process, we must briefly examine the dominant conceptual models that historically have formed the basis for consultation-liaison psychiatry.

In Western medical practice, the clinical practice of consultation-liaison psychiatry is inextricably tied to historical developments in psychosomatic medicine and experimental psychophysiology. Recent works on the history of clinical consultation-liaison psychiatry authored by Dr. J. Schwab (1989) and Dr. Z. J. Lipowski (1986a), as well as several others (Hackett 1987; Kimball 1970; Kollar and Alcalay 1967; Lipowski 1986b; Summergrad and Hackett 1987), offer a variety of perspectives on this highly specialized and interesting topic.

Historically, physicians and nonphysicians alike have recognized the important role played by the mind in the initiation, presentation, and/or course of medical illness (Ackernecht 1982). While greatly admired physicians (Osler 1943; Rush 1811) have advised their students to attend to such factors in their medical practice, only in the past half-century has the profession systematically incorporated psychological factors into medical practice.

Most historical accounts of the development of consultation-liaison psychiatry address the psychosomatic medicine tradition and, more recently, the role of the liaison. However, several other modalities have contributed significantly to the clinical base of consultation-liaison psychiatry. For example, the clinical base of consultation-liaison psychiatry has been altered by advances in general psychiatry, brief and crisis-oriented psychotherapy, behavioral medicine, systems theory, biological psychiatry, neuropsychology, and behavioral neurology. This list of contributions reflects the role of consultation-liaison as a synthetic discipline. In turn, this synthetic character renders a historical treatise on consultation-liaison psychiatry beyond the scope of this book. Despite this constraint, however, we will provide a brief overview of how consultation-liaison psychiatry and its most closely related scientific field, psychosomatic medicine, developed. For quick reference, we also provide an appendix summarizing significant events in this history.

Historical Overview of Consultation-Liaison Clinical Practice

Consultation-liaison psychiatry originated in America in the mid-1700s. Early practice was rooted in certain clinically astute physicians' belief that the mind and body are inextricably linked. In the twentieth century, the consultation-liaison subspecialty developed more quickly as psychiatric departments began to open in general hospitals (as opposed to free-standing clinics [Kaufman 1965]).

World War I further invigorated the clinical practice of consultation-liaison psychiatry. This is a period that saw nearly 50,000 men rejected from the military because of nervous and mental disorders and 72,000 inductees discharged from the service because of neuropsychiatric conditions (Ireland 1923). The psychiatric casualties of World War II accounted for 23% of all evacuations in contrast to 7% for Vietnam (Ursano and Holloway 1985).

In the 1930s and 1940s, the expansion of educational programs triggered further growth in consultation-liaison programs; research activities and special training for psychiatric residents and medical students (Schwab 1989) followed. In 1934, for example, the Rockefeller Foundation funded five university hospital-based psychiatric-liaison departments (Lipowski 1986a). Additionally, many credit Dr. James Eaton of the National Institute of Mental Health's (NIMH) Psychiatry Education Branch for powerfully influencing the development of the specialty. Under his aegis in the 1970s and 1980s, over 100 programs and several hundred fellows received support for consultation-liaison activities from this NIMH branch (Eaton et al. 1977; Lipowski 1986a). More recently, programs and research have grown more slowly (Schwab 1989), and monetary pressures have led to the restructuring of existing programs (see Chapter 12). While early consultation-liaison programs were well subsidized, reimbursement has become more difficult and less reliable (Fenton 1981).

Despite these setbacks, the profession continues to fortify the role of consultation-liaison in medical treatment. First, and most importantly, the scientific base for its practice has been widened. A past half-century of progress in psychobiology now solidly grounds the clinical practice of consultation-liaison psychiatry in the general hospital. However, the spirit of consultation-liaison psychiatry remains in its commitment to working collaboratively with nonpsychiatric caregivers about the psychiatric management of their patients. Thus, successful consultations often entail managing complex or crisis situations on medical wards—a role central to the subspecialty. While most other medical subspecialties have analogous consultation teams, physicians in these teams play a role that is considerably more limited and conceptually more simple than the role of the consultation-liaison psychiatrist. Currently, a lively debate is taking place over how to establish consultation-liaison as a subspecialty area of practice (Pasnau 1988; Yager and Langsley 1987). In response to this debate, supporters have justified consultation-liaison's role in the health-care system on the grounds that it is cost-effective (see Chapter 12; Pincus 1984) and an effectively marketable product (Wise 1987).

Historical Developments in Scientific Theories of Psychobiology

Traditionally, the consultation-liaison psychiatrist has been interested in the changes in physiology and the course of illness as affected by psychosocial factors (psychosomatic medicine). Indeed, differentiating the varying contributions of psychosocial factors and medical disease requires considerable collaboration between the general medical physician and the psychiatrist. Thus, the history of consultation-liaison psychiatry and the history of theories of psychobiology are inseparably connected.

In the past decades many articles (see Ackernecht 1982; Lipowski 1986b; Wise 1986; Meyes 1951 for reviews) and books have addressed the psychobiology of human disease. Weiner's noteworthy book (1977), for example, reviews the scientific basis for the current psychobiological models of specific diseases that are considered to be significantly affected by psychological factors (peptic ulcer, asthma, Graves' disease, rheumatoid arthritis, essential hypertension, and ulcerative colitis). Weiner stresses the important interactions among multiple levels of psychological and biological factors in the etiology of all these illnesses.

These recent conceptualizations stem from earlier studies based first on anecdotal observations and later on animal research and careful scientific methodology. The traditional conceptions of psychosomatics envisioned emotions, often specific intrapsychic conflicts (Alexander 1950), as causing particular diseases. Developed from classic descriptions by Dr. William Beaumont in the early 1800s, this theory recognized that emotions profoundly affected autonomic physiology. Beaumont observed that emotions, such as anger, in a wounded soldier dramatically changed gastric secretion, motility, and blood engorgement in a segment of exposed bowel mucosa.

Prior to the twentieth century, however, studies of the relationship between emotions and body function continued to be limited to isolated observations. In this century, investigation into the mind-body link has been enriched by an explosion of information derived from the systematization of scientific methods and more extensive animal research.

Performed by Cannon (1920, 1932), Pavlov, and Selye (1936, 1956), early animal studies provided the foundation for the way we now conceptualize psychosomatic interactions. These studies enabled later researchers to design experimental models that have furthered the development of consultation-liaison as a subspecialty area of practice.

An American researcher working with natural reactions in cats, Cannon demonstrated fight/flight reactions, with their attendant dramatic changes in physiology. Pavlov, a Russian scientist, documented the way autonomic responses could be "conditioned" in dogs, that is, how an experimenter could manipulate and predictively control those responses. Today, Pavlov's work has been extended to the modern biofeedback control of such functions as brain waves, blood flow, skin temperature, etc., and his theoretical base underlies much current behavioral medicine (Garrick 1989).

Another early researcher, Selye, an Austrian-Canadian, introduced the concept of biological stress (Selye 1936) and identified and performed an extraordinary number of studies on the physiology of responses to various stressors. Unlike Cannon, who emphasized the catecholamine response to stressors, Selye underscored the importance of the pituitary-adrenal axis and corticoid hormones in modulating stress reactions and the pathological responses to chronic stress. Selye emphasized the nonspecificity of the body's stress reactions and noted organ failure resulting from chronic stress.

While Selye's work is still valid today, additional research has demonstrated that a greater organ specificity underlies many psychophysiological responses. For example, in a classic study performed in 1957, Weiner and his colleagues were able to differentiate, on the basis of psychological data alone, those persons who secreted large amounts of gastric acid from those who secreted very little. Using a battery of psychological tests and monitoring blood pepsinogen levels, Weiner was able to predict nearly half of the army recruits who developed duodenal ulcers during basic training. Working from the early animal and human research, Weiner and others derived the foundation for the later biopsychosocial models of disease by stressing that biological, psychological, and social factors interact to cause disease. Today, the concept "psychosomatic reaction" refers to a complex combination of biological and psychosocial factors, all of which contribute to the onset, maintenance, and expression of most diseases. Engel (1977, 1982) described this concept most clearly with his biopsychosocial model of disease.

Translating these physiological findings (both theoretical and practical) into clinical practice has been difficult. The appendix outlines the conceptual development of our understanding (in Western science) of these important illnesses, a topic that overlaps the growth of the larger field of psychiatry itself. If the articulation of psychosomatic concepts has been the greatest influence on how consultation-liaison psychiatry has developed, further advances in the field will continue to be intimately linked to our capacity to clarify both the precise mediating mechanisms of brain-body physiology and the molecular biology of these functions.

REFERENCES

Abram HS: Adaptation to open heart surgery: a psychiatric study of response to the threat of death. Am J Psychiatry 122:659–668, 1965

Ackernecht EH: The history of psychosomatic medicine. Psychol Med 12:17–24, 1982

Adamson JD, Schmale AH: Object loss, giving up and the onset of psychiatric disease. Psychosom Med 27:557–576, 1965

Ader R, Cohen N: Behaviorally conditioned immunosuppression. Psychosom Med 37:333–340, 1975

Alexander F: Psychosomatic Medicine. New York, WW Norton, 1950

Beebe JE III, Rosenbaum CP: Outpatient therapy: an overview, in Psychiatric Treatment. Edited by Rosenbaum CP, Beebe JE III. New York, McGraw-Hill, 1975, pp 227–263

Bridger WH, Reiser MF: Psychophysiologic studies of the neonate: an approach toward the methodological and theoretical problems involved. Psychosom Med 21:265–276, 1959

Cannon WB: Bodily Changes in Pain, Hunger, Fear and Rage. New York, Appleton, 1920

Cannon WB: The Wisdom of the Body. New York, WW Norton, 1932

Cleghorn RA, Graham BF: Studies of adrenal cortical activity in psychoneurotic subjects. Am J Psychiatry 106:668–672, 1950

Dunbar HF: Emotions and Bodily Changes: A Survey of Literature on Psychosomatic Interrelationships. New York, Columbia University Press, 1954

Eaton JS, Goldberg R, Rosinski E, et al: The educational challenge of consultation-liaison psychiatry. Am J Psychiatry 134:20–23, 1977

Engel GL: A life setting conducive to illness: the giving up–given up complex. Bull Menninger Clin 32:355–365, 1960

Engel GL: A reconsideration of the role of conversion in somatic disease. Compr Psychiatry 9:316–326, 1968

Engel GL: The need for a new medical model: a challenge for biomedicine. Science 196:129–136, 1977

Engel GL: The bio-psychosocial model and medical education: who are to be the teachers? N Engl J Med 13:802–805, 1982

Fava GA, Trombini G, Grandi S, et al: A psychosomatic outpatient clinic. Int J Psychiatry Med 17:261–267, 1987

Fenton BJ, Guggenheim FG: Consultation-liaison psychiatry and funding: why can't Alice find Wonderland? Gen Hosp Psychiatry 7:255–260, 1981

Fras I, Litin EM, Bartholomew LG: Mental symptoms as an aid in the early diagnosis of carcinoma of the pancreas. Gastroenterology 55:191–197, 1968

Freyberger H, Kunsebeck H, Lempa W, et al: The Hannover consultation liaison model: some empirical findings. Soc Sci Med 21:1391–1404, 1985

Friedman M, Rosenman RH: Association of specific overt behavior pattern with blood and cardiovascular findings. JAMA 169:1286–1296, 1959

Funkenstein DH, King SH, Drolette M: Mastery of Stress. Cambridge, MA, Harvard University Press, 1957

Garrick T, Loewenstein R: Behavioral medicine in the general hospital. Psychosomatics 30:123–134, 1989

Graham DT, Lundy RM, Benjamin LS, et al: Specific attitudes in initial interviews with patients having different "psychosomatic" diseases. Psychosom Med 24:257–266, 1962

Greene WA Jr: Preliminary observations on a group of males with lymphomas and leukemias. Psychosom Med 16:220–230, 1954

Greene WA Jr: Some perspectives for observing and interpreting biopsychologic relation and doctor-patient relations. Perspect Biol Med 2:453–472, 1959

Greene WA Jr, Young LE, Swisher SN: Psychological factors and reticulo-endothelial disease. II. Observations on a group of women with lymphomas and leukemias. Psychosom Med 18:284–303, 1956

Grinker RR, Robbins FP: Psychosomatic Case Book. New York, Blakiston, 1954

Hackett TP: Beginnings: consultation psychiatry in a general hospital, in Massachusetts General Hospital Handbook of General Hospital Psychiatry, 2nd Edition. Edited by Hackett TP, Cassem NH. Littleton, MA, PSG Publishers, 1987, pp 1–13

Hamburg AD, Adams JE: A perspective on coping behavior. Arch Gen Psychiatry 17:277–284, 1967

Hinkle LE, Wolf S: A summary of experimental evidence relating life stress to diabetes mellitus. J Mt Sinai Hosp 19:537–570, 1952

Hohman GW: Some effects of spinal cord lesions in experienced emotional feelings. Psychophysiology 3:143–156, 1966

Holmes TH, Rahe RH: The social readjustment scale. J Psychosom Res 11:213–218, 1967

Ireland GO: The neuro-psychiatric ex-serviceman and his civil re-establishment. Am J Psychiatry 2:685–711, 1923

Iwasaka T: Teaching liaison psychiatry and clinical practice of psychosomatic medicine in the general hospital, in The Teaching of Psychosomatic Medicine and Consultation-Liaison Psychiatry. Edited by Kimball CP, Krakowski AJ. Bibliotheca Psychiatrica, No 159. Basel, S Karger, 1979, pp 32–38

Kaufman MR: The Psychiatric Unit in a General Hospital. New York, International Universities Press, 1965

Kimball CP: Conceptual developments in psychosomatic medicine; 1939–1969. Ann Intern Med 73:307–316, 1970

Kimball CP (ed): Psychiatric Clinics of North America, Vol 2, No 2. Philadelphia, PA, WB Saunders, 1979

Kollar EJ, Alcalay M: The physiological basis for psychosomatic medicine. A historical view. Ann Intern Med 67:883–895, 1967

Levitan S, Kornfeld D: Clinical and cost benefits of liaison psychiatry. Am J Psychiatry 138:790–793, 1981

Lipowski ZJ: Consultation-liaison psychiatry: past, present and future, in Consultation-Liaison Psychiatry. Edited by Pasnau RO. New York, Grune & Stratton, 1975, pp 1–30

Lipowski ZJ: Consultation-liaison psychiatry: the first half century. Gen Hosp Psychiatry 8:305–315, 1986a

Lipowski ZJ: Psychosomatic medicine: past and present. Part 1. Historical background. Can J Psychiatry 31:2–7, 1986b

Lyons JS, Hammer JS, Strain JJ, et al: The timing of psychiatric consultation in the general hospital and length of hospital stay. Gen Hosp Psychiatry 8:159–162, 1986

Mason JW: The scope of psychoendocrine research. Psychosom Med 30:565–575, 1968

Meyer A: The psychobiological point of view, in The Collected Papers of Adolf Meyer, Vol 3, Medical Teaching. Edited by Winters EE. Baltimore, MD, Johns Hopkins University Press, 1951, pp 429–443

Miller NE: Learning of visceral and glandular responses. Science 163:434–445, 1969

Mumford E, Schlesinger H, Glass G, et al: A new look at evidence about reduced cost of medical utilization following medical treatment. Am J Psychiatry 141:1145–1158, 1984

Osler W: Aequanimitas. Philadelphia, PA, Blakiston, 1943

Pasnau RO (ed): Consultation-Liaison Psychiatry. New York, Grune & Stratton, 1975

Pasnau RO: Consultation-liaison psychiatry: progress, problems and prospects. Psychosomatics 29:4–15, 1988

Pincus HA: Making the case for consultation-liaison psychiatry: issues in cost-effectiveness analysis. Gen Hosp Psychiatry 6:173–179, 1984

Ruesch J: The infantile personality. Psychosom Med 10:134–144, 1948

Rush B: Sixteen Introductory Lectures. Philadelphia, PA, Bradford and Innskeep, 1811

Schmale AH Jr: Relationship of separation and depression to disease: I. A report on a hospitalized medical population. Psychosom Med 20:259–277, 1958

Schwab J: Consultation-liaison psychiatry: a historical overview. Psychosomatics 30:245–254, 1989

Schwab JJ, Bialow M, Brown JM, et al: Diagnosing depression in medical inpatients. Ann Intern Med 67:695–707, 1967

Schwartz J, Speed N, Kuskowski M: A psychiatric consultation/liaison clinic: follow-up of fifty-four patients referred from neurology. Int J Psychiatry Med 17:213–221, 1987

Selye H: Syndrome produced by diverse noxious agents. Nature 138: 32–40, 1936

Selye H: The Physiology and Pathology of Exposure to Stress. Montreal, Acta, 1950

Selye H: The Stress of Life. New York, McGraw-Hill, 1956

Sontag LW, Wallace RF: Preliminary report of the Fels Fund: study of fetal activity. Am J Dis Child 48:1050–1057, 1934

Stein M, Schiavi R, Camierino M: Influence of brain and behavior in the immune system. Science 191:435–440, 1976

Steinhilber RM, Peterson HW Jr, Martin MJ: Emotional states caused by organic diseases. Postgrad Med 39:621–630, 1966

Strain JJ, Grossman S: Psychological Care of the Medically Ill. New York, Appleton-Century-Crofts, 1975

Summergrad P, Hackett TP: Alan Gregg and the rise of general hospital psychiatry. Gen Hosp Psychiatry 9:439–445, 1987

Ursano RJ, Holloway HC: Military psychiatry, in Comprehensive Textbook of Psychiatry, 4th Edition, Vol 2. Edited by Kaplan HI, Sadock BJ. Baltimore, MD, Williams & Wilkins, 1985, pp 1900–1909

Weiner H: Psychobiology and Human Disease. New York, Elsevier North-Holland, 1977

Weiner H, Thaler M, Reiser MF, et al: Etiology of duodenal ulcer. Psychosom Med 19:1–10, 1957

Wise TN: Psychosomatic medicine: integrating dynamic, behavioral and biological perspectives. Psychother Psychosom 46:85–95, 1986

Wise TN: Segmenting and accessing the market in consultation-liaison psychiatry. Gen Hosp Psychiatry 9:354–359, 1987

Wolcott DL, Fawzey FI, Pasnau RO: Consultation-liaison outpatient clinics. Gen Hosp Psychiatry 6:153–161, 1984

Wolff HG: Stress and Disease. Springfield, IL, Charles C Thomas, 1953

Yager J, Langsley DG: The evolving subspecialization of psychiatry: implications for the profession. Am J Psychiatry 144:1461–1465, 1987

Appendix: Conceptual History of Psychosomatic Medicine[1]

I. Early Observations on Effect of Emotions on Physiology

A. Ancient observations: Emotions cause physiologic alterations, medical illness, and bodily disease (Ackernecht 1982; Steinhilber et al. 1966).

B. Cannon (1920) systematically showed that fight/flight reactions change autonomic functioning. Formulated the concept of "homeostasis," which provided the foundation for a holistic view of mind-body functioning (Kollar and Alcalay 1967).

C. Funkenstein, King, and Drolette (1957) demonstrated that epinephrine mimics reactions of anger.

D. Selye (1950) suggested that adaptive reactions may lead to disease because they upset the internal balance of the body. He also found that chronic biological stress causes organ failure.

II. Somatopsychic Correlations

Several disease states have been shown to affect or be associated with emotional status:

A. Frontal-lobe meningioma has been associated with suicidal behavior.
B. Pancreatic cancer has been associated with depression (Fras et al. 1968).
C. Temporal-lobe astrocytoma has been associated with delusions.
D. Hypoglycemia (secondary to pancreatic adenoma) may induce psychosis.
E. Hyperthyroidism may induce agitated depression.
F. Pheochromocytoma may induce anxiety.
G. Pernicious anemia may induce depression and apathy.
H. Wilson's disease may induce behavioral disturbance.
I. Addison's disease may induce fatigue.
J. Cushing's disease may induce euphoria and depression.
K. Delirium caused by multiple illnesses.

---

[1] Adapted from Kimball 1970.

III. Personality-Illness Specificity

A. Personality specificity (Dunbar 1954): certain personality characteristics are thought to be associated with certain disease types.

B. An infantile personality is posited by Ruesch (1948) to be the core problem in all psychosomatic patients.

C. Friedman and Rosenman (1959): Type A personality is identified as predisposing toward heart disease in both retrospective and prospective studies.

IV. Conflict-Onset Situation

A. Alexander and French (Alexander 1948) identify the "holy seven" psychosomatic diseases: hyperthyroidism, neurodermatitis, peptic ulcer, rheumatoid arthritis, essential hypertension, bronchial asthma, and ulcerative colitis. Specific conflicts are thought to predispose certain individuals to develop each illness in the context of specific organ vulnerability (e.g., genetic weakness).

B. Weiner and Mirsky (Weiner et al. 1957) prospectively demonstrated the production of duodenal ulcer in individuals with elevated pepsinogen levels and specific psychological characteristics.

C. Wolff (1953) used stressful interviews with conflict-laden material to elicit physiological changes in specific organs.

D. Hinkle and Wolf (1952) demonstrated that control of blood sugar in diabetic patients relates to life experiences, conflicts, and coping abilities.

V. Individual Physiological Specificity

A. Sontag and Wallace (1934) and Bridger and Reiser (1959) demonstrated specific, longitudinally consistent individual variations in autonomic reactivity in response to mild stress in fetuses.

VI. Illness-Onset Situation

A. Holmes and Rahe (1967; Rahe, manuscripts in preparation) defined a series of life stresses that, when experienced in an additive fashion, strongly predisposed to disease in a specific time period following the experiences.

VII. General Systems Theory

A. Grinker and Robbins (1954), Cleghorn and Graham (1950), Hamburg and Adams (1967), and Mason (1968) identified adaptive processes correlated with adrenal cortical activity. These processes relate to a wide variety of psychosocial needs rather than to any specific one.

VIII. Object Loss, Affect State, and Illness

A. Greene (1954, 1959) and colleagues (Greene et al. 1956) identified premorbid personalities common to patients with lymphomas, leukemia, and Hodgkin's disease, and the proximity of object loss to the disease onset. Others confirmed the relationship of object loss to disease onset (Adamson 1965; Schmale 1958).

B. Engel (1960, 1968) identifies the giving-up–given-up complex related to physiological hypoactivity and the onset of both psychiatric and somatic disease.

IX. Adaptation

A. Schwab (1967) identified "somatopsychic" relationships in medically ill patients in which the individual has various response patterns (grief/depression, anxiety/denial, changed self concept, disturbed interpersonal relationships).

B. The course of a wide variety of illnesses (e.g., diabetes [Graham et al. 1962]), procedures (e.g., surgery [Abram 1965]), dying, chronic disease, and permanent physical impairment (e.g., paraplegia [Hohman 1966]) is affected by the person's coping strategies.

X. Behavioral Effects on Physiology

A. Miller (1969) documents that autonomic functions can be operantly conditioned in animals, leading the way to the development of biofeedback, meditation, and relaxation training.

B. Specific behavioral and operant effects on immune function (Ader and Cohen 1975; Stein and Schiavi 1976) suggest specific mediating mechanisms for how stress causes physiological and anatomic dysfunction.

2

Setting the Stage

This chapter outlines the steps for introducing a psychiatric consultation service in a new setting, or making major changes in procedures or personnel in an existing service. The history of psychiatric consultation and liaison summarized in the previous chapter will have given the reader some introduction to the various collaborative styles that have evolved. Psychiatric involvement in general hospital practice can range from occasional lectures to regularly scheduled teaching, from responses to rare and urgent referrals to daily rounding on all patients. By "consultation service" we mean any structured arrangement whereby psychiatric opinions and recommendations with respect to hospital inpatients are obtained. The outline is general and can be adapted to meet the needs and utilize the resources of a variety of clinical settings. The word "unit," as used below, means any identified organization to which the psychiatrist will be a consultant: a hospital floor or other geographic area, a specialty or subspecialty service, or a patient-care team.

Consulting in a New Setting

Some hospital inpatient units have no formal setting for obtaining psychiatric assessments and care for patients who need them.

The need for such a system may be identified by the primary attending physicians, by other staff members caring for patients, or by an individual psychiatrist or psychiatry department aware of the unmet need. Before setting up the specific procedures for a new consultation service, the psychiatrist must understand the system of which this service will be a part (Schwab 1968). The following questions are relevant to an understanding of the system:

1. What personnel constitute the patient-care system?
2. Why has there been no, or a different, psychiatric consultation arrangement? Is the need for one perceived by the potential consultees? If so, are they unanimous or divided in their opinions?
3. Has there been an unsatisfactory experience in the past? If so, what was it?
4. What are the attitudes of the primary physicians toward psychiatry? (Psychiatry, as a specialty, probably evokes more affect and conflict than any other specialty [Hawkins 1962].)
5. What are the practice patterns of the primary physicians and the unit?
   To what medical specialty, if any, is the unit devoted?
6. What patient population does the hospital or unit serve?
7. How do these patients pay for their care? How will consultations be funded?
8. How is the unit organized?
9. What are the educational needs and programs of the unit?

The potential consultant will want to know not only the unit's formal structure but also its "character" and unwritten rules. Proposing a consultation arrangement requires great sensitivity to territorial feelings and to anxieties about the disruption of comfortable, established practice patterns and the possible exposure of ignorance about psychiatric issues (Lipowski 1967). The psychiatrist is an unknown (Mohl 1977).

Meeting the Staff

A consultation service cannot exist without the permission—whether enthusiastic, passive, or reluctant—of the primary physicians responsible for patients. The primary physicians rarely object to the idea in principle. (Working with them will be described in the next chapter.) But many other members of the hospital staff are also crucial to the consultation process. It is a worthwhile investment to meet them, learn about their roles and functions on the unit, elicit their concerns about the system in general and about psychiatric consultation in particular, and become familiar with their characters and patient-care styles.

Administrators

Hospital and unit administrators are responsible for aspects of patient care crucial to psychiatric consultation. They may make rules about visiting concerning, for example, visiting hours; numbers, relationships, and ages of visitors allowed; whether "significant others" may sleep in the patient's room, etc. Administrators are often called when patients wish to sign out against medical advice, refuse strongly advised procedures, or insist on deviations from hospital policies such as removal of newborn babies to the nursery. In addition, they have access to, and are experts on, information about patients' medical insurance coverage.

These issues relate to psychiatric consultation in at least three ways: (a) access of patients to care in general and their psychological responses to medical and/or financial problems, (b) questions concerning length of stay, and (c) coverage for psychiatric consultation and recommended inpatient and/or outpatient psychiatric care. A brief office meeting or informal lunch will serve to demonstrate the respect and interest of the new psychiatric consultant, allow for the exchange of ideas and the mutual observation of styles, enhance credibility, and offer an opportunity for the airing of questions and concerns. A working relationship with the administrator(s) can forestall problems and facilitate collaboration when any of the above issues enters into a patient's care.

Secretaries/Clerks

On many units, secretaries or clerks are responsible for ordering and arranging tests and consultations for patients. They know everyone on the unit and have an overview of unit function. They also deal with people who telephone the floor and visit patients. A clerk who has met and feels friendly toward a consultant is more likely to persist in trying to make contact when the consultant is not immediately available. The clerk can help the consultant contact the members of the attending, house, nursing, and other staffs who were responsible for asking for the consultation and/or who know the patient best. The clerk is often most aware of scheduled radiographic examinations and other procedures that may take the patient away from the floor, and other aspects of unit schedules, such as mealtimes and rounding times, the knowledge of which facilitates the contact of the consultant with patient and staff. The secretary can locate an elusive hospital chart and see to it that consultation notes are entered into it in a timely and accessible way. A clerk who knows the consultant can relay an important message.

In general, familiarity with the permanent staff integrates the consultant into the unit in a tangible and comfortable way. Getting to know the unit secretary's name and making a point of extending a greeting and exchanging pleasantries on visits to the unit foster that end.

Social Workers

In many settings, social workers are the main or only psychosocial resource for patients and their health-care providers. Awareness of the social workers' practice patterns, and of the demands and constraints upon these workers, is essential to consistent, comprehensive care.

The relationship between psychiatry and social work exemplifies and highlights the "turf battles" and quest for professional identity and boundaries that characterize the relationships between mental health professionals. The task for a new consultation-liaison psychiatrist may range from the performance of services for which medical social workers are unavailable in the setting, to demonstrating a need for and recruiting social work staff, to dealing with the resentment of social workers who have provided all of the psychosocial assessment, treatment, and referral services on a unit for years.

Upon introduction to a new unit, ascertain who, if anyone, has been monitoring patients' adaptation to illness, psychological symptoms and signs, family and social supports, and plans for discharge. If there is not a social service consultant available who is knowledgeable about community resources such as visiting nurses, convalescent facilities, home-care services, hospices, counseling and mental health centers, and who is conversant with the intricacies of the state and federal health and disability coverage plans, a psychiatrist may be either handicapped in arranging comprehensive patient care or burdened with tasks for which he or she is neither trained nor compensated. Perhaps the consultation arrangement should be made contingent upon the provision of social work collaboration.

Where there are social workers assigned to the unit, meet with them to learn what they have been doing, how they view their roles, and what their concerns about and expectations for psychiatric consultation are. Allow them to get to know and feel comfortable with you and the process by which you are formulating a plan for consultation services. In many major medical centers, recent financial cutbacks have resulted in decreases in social work staffing. The remaining social workers often are overworked and painfully aware of their inability to meet desperate patient needs.

The situation is complicated by pressures to shorten hospital stays and rigorously account for the medical necessity of bed utilization. Thus, a reduced number of social workers must tend to patients who are more ill when admitted and more disabled when discharged. Often, patients and their families must be prepared to deal with tracheostomies, oxygen machines, ambulatory dialysis, indwelling catheters, and/or artificial routes of nourishment, as well as impaired capacity to ambulate. To complicate matters still further, many procedures are performed on an outpatient basis, so that sick patients must be conveyed back and forth from home to the medical facility. Social workers must make increasing numbers of these arrangements with decreasing lead time. The availability of psychiatric consultation may be perceived as a resource and/or as an additional complication.

The information helpful to the potential consultant is obtained by answering the following questions:

- For what units is the social worker responsible?
- What are the average and ranges of patient census for each unit, the hours the social worker is available, and the allotment of his or her time among outpatient, administrative, bedside, family, and other duties?

- Does the social worker follow any patients after discharge?
- What is the best time to call or meet with the social worker, and how may he or she be reached? (The social worker will also want to know how to reach you.)

This raises another issue. Generally, consultation among medical practitioners is formally initiated by the patient's primary physician; it is a service offered by one physician to another (Lipowski 1974). Many health-care plans and third-party payers require that specialty consultations be ordered by a referring physician. However, some social workers, units, and psychiatric consultants may find it preferable or simply realistic to empower social workers, as mental health professionals, to identify the need for and initiate psychiatric consultations.

Practices vary from service to service and from hospital to hospital. The social worker, the patient, or the nursing or house staff may set the process in motion, while the primary or attending physician signs the written request. The procedure should be clear, consistent, practical, and comfortable to all concerned.

Psychologists and Other Mental Health Professionals

Similar situations arise with other mental health professionals: psychologists, nurse clinicians and specialists, behavioral medicine specialists, and pastoral counselors. In each case, areas of responsibility, hierarchies of authority, referral procedures in both directions, and logistics must be delineated. In most cases, a shared interest in patients' welfare facilitates a mutually workable solution. However, ethical, legal, and medical responsibility for patients' psychophysiological, emotional, and behavioral well-being will tend to rest with the psychiatrist, who is a physician. The decision-making and referral process settled upon must take this reality into account.

The functions of psychologists in a general hospital setting fall into several categories. Sometimes they are the only, or main, resource for psychological assessment and care. Sometimes they specialize in so-called "behavioral medicine," using behavioral modification techniques to deal with clinical problems such as pain, anxiety, noncompliance, and other issues (Abel et al. 1987). Because psychiatrists are specialists in the interrelatedness of behavior and medical illness, the designation of "behavioral medicine" as a subspecialty of psychology is a subject of controversy. Cognitive and behavioral treatments, such as distraction, relaxation, sensate focus exercises, etc., are also learned and practiced by psychiatrists who find them useful in work with the medically ill.

Psychologists may provide psychological and neuropsychological testing services that are an important component of psychiatric assessment and care for patients at risk for organic brain disease (Fogel and Faust 1987). An expert neuropsychologist can often diagnose the nature and location of a central nervous system (CNS) lesion. A psychiatrist planning to offer consultation to a unit serving many patients at risk for such lesions might want to ensure that such a neuropsychologist is available for collaboration.

The relationship between the psychiatric consultation service and the psychologist, if any, depends upon which of the above roles the psychologist has fulfilled. If the unit to which you will consult has been working with a psychologist, read a representative sample of the reports provided. Do they include a full mental status examination and a complete personal, family, and social history? Does the psychologist address the possibility that the patient's symptoms are related to pharmacologic treatment for the primary disease, metabolic derangements, and/or physical illness? Is there a full differential diagnosis? Are the recommended interventions appropriate and comprehensive?

Administrators, nonpsychiatric physicians, and managed health plans may operate under the misconception that nonmedical mental health professionals can assess and manage "psychological" or "emotional" aspects of patients' illnesses while the primary physician sees to the "medical" aspects. Such an arrangement does not take into account the complex interrelations between "psyche" and "soma" that are intrinsic to all illness (Engel 1977).

You will want to meet with the psychologist to discuss approaches to consultation, theoretical orientation, experience, and styles of work. If you are to share responsibility, you must feel comfortable that your approaches and expertise are compatible with those of the psychologist. If you are to supervise and refer to the psychologist, you need to know what work you can delegate. Should you have serious concerns about the current level of service, you must be able to support them with data.

Nursing Staff

Nursing is another profession in the process of redefining its identity and its relationship with other health-care providers. Many nurses have become disenchanted with the role of hand-maiden to physicians and have fought for increased autonomy and authority. A shortage of bedside nurses has developed as potential students choose other fields and trained nurses seek advanced training in nursing or related areas. Many hospitals have vice presidents for or clinical chiefs of nursing, so that nurses answer to their own administrators rather than to physicians.

Nurses justifiably stress their function and expertise as the staff who spend the most time at the bedside. They acquire detailed information on the patient's personality and response to illness and treatment. They often learn which management style works best with each patient. They observe and interact with family and other visitors and may note the effect of their visits on the patient's mental status.

Each hospital unit has its own pattern of, and problems with, nursing care. Many units are understaffed. A psychiatric consultant who suggests additional complex tasks and/or alienates nurses will not be well regarded. Nurses' overwork and inability to live up to their own high standards for patient care are frustrating and demoralizing, especially when coupled with increasing amounts of paperwork and the need to master complex technical procedures. Understaffing often results in shifts of assignments, so that nurses on a unit may be unfamiliar both with its procedures and with its patients. The latter problem is further complicated by shortened hospital stays. The practice of "primary nursing," by which a specific nurse is assigned to care for and coordinate the needs of specific patients throughout their hospital stays, is an attempt to address these problems.

On some specialized units, highly trained nurses handle extremely intricate, physically, emotionally, and intellectually demanding skills such as dialysis and cardiac monitoring. Often they are far more knowledgeable and adept than the members of the house or general medical staff who issue the orders. Their need to train physicians may be acknowledged and appreciated, or surreptitious. These nurses also become familiar with the experiences and behaviors of patients undergoing a particular illness or treatment, such as a burn or coronary bypass surgery.

The psychiatric consultant needs to know what the nursing situation on the consultee unit is, and to develop a strong working relationship with the nursing staff (Mohl 1984). It is the nurse who can chart the hour-by-hour or minute-by-minute response of the patient to psychotropic or analgesic medication, carefully document sleep and eating behaviors, notate crucial patient statements (e.g., "There are bugs crawling on my skin," "Sometimes I think I will jump out the window," "They are sending me a special message through the television"), and/or observe whether symptoms and behaviors are consistent under a variety of circumstances (e.g., patient cannot walk when the medical service makes rounds, but gets up to fetch forbidden cigarettes from the other side of the room).

Nurses are often interested in continuing education in psychiatric issues, and in individual and/or group support in difficult cases, such as the death of a patient who had become particularly close to the staff or a patient experienced as "impossible." Teaching conferences are an excellent opportunity to demonstrate the psychiatric consultant's competence, interest, and availability, while the consultant can learn the styles and needs of the nursing staff. Often it is nurses who alert the medical staff or consultant to the changing, aberrant, or problematic behavior of patients who will benefit from psychiatric consultation. In some settings, specialized nurses are a key part of the consultation-liaison psychiatry team (O'Connor and Bilodeau 1987). In others, psychiatric liaison nurses function independently to advise fellow nurses on patient-care units. The psychiatric consultant can do much to foster the recognition and integration of nursing contributions to patients' biopsychosocial care.

Other Specialized Service Staff

Hospital staffs include specialized care providers of a variety of disciplines. Some, like X-ray technicians, have brief and sporadic contact with patients and are not critical to the patients' psychosocial care unless there is a major problem of some sort. Others, like respiratory therapists, interact frequently and consistently with many patients, but usually in a nonindividualized way. Still others, such as physical and occupational therapists, speech therapists, nutritionists, and educators who teach patients about specific diseases and treatments (e.g., diabetes, ambulatory peritoneal dialysis, sexual life after myocardial infarction), are centrally involved with patients' psychological conditions.

Like nurses, these staff members can help the psychiatric consultant with knowledge about typical responses to illness and detailed observations about patients' adaptations, and can sometimes use suggestions from the consultant for understanding and working with patients. Find out who works on the unit where you will consult, what services they offer, what questions and needs they have, and how best to get in touch with them. If there are frequently used ancillary-care locations, such as a dialysis center, whirlpool, radiation therapy area, or rehabilitation center, visit them and observe the staff and patients using them.

Members of the Clergy

Religious resources may be overlooked in the practice of psychiatry. Patients undergoing the rigors of medical illness and treatment may derive significant solace from religious beliefs and members of the clergy. At other times, their suffering interferes with their faith, deepening their consternation, alienation, and desolation. They feel angry at and deserted by the divine being they most need for comfort. In many hospitals, there are chaplains on the staff, available to address the spiritual needs of patients and their families. The chaplains may be Christian but otherwise nondenominational, or there may be a variety of clergy on call for patients of particular religious affiliations.

Oftentimes chaplains call on patients routinely to offer support. (Some patients feel uncomfortable or annoyed about this; the psychiatric consultant might help by indicating, at the patient's request, that further visits are not desired.) Chaplains may call specifically on those patients who indicated a particular religious affiliation during the process of admission to the hospital. The psychiatric consultant who is informed about the available religious resources can call upon them to help a patient or family member pained by a theological question (e.g., "Would an abortion in my current circumstances invoke divine punishment?"), interested in a religious ritual (e.g., burial of a stillborn child, last rites for the dying, baptism), or desirous of a leader or partner in prayer.

House Staff

As members of the house staff rotate among hospital services, it is necessary to introduce oneself to a new team on most units every month or so. House officers tend to be wary of activities that may entail additions to their already heavy workload, especially when psychosocial matters are not perceived as a priority of the attending staff who control their schedules and their evaluations. They are also understandably anxious, manifestly or latently, about the revelation of any lack of expertise or thoroughness in patient care (Adler 1972).

Trainees, who are still in their formative years of medical practice, are worthy of considerable educational effort. Some will be relieved to share their questions and problems, while others will treat psychiatrists with a distaste presumably learned from their role models in medical school and residency. The offering of consultation as a genuinely helpful resource will have to be both stated and demonstrated. (Suggestions for specific modes of interaction are discussed later in this chapter.)

ESTABLISHING THE CONSULTANT-CONSULTEE RELATIONSHIP

While, for all the reasons stated, it is critical to get to know all the staff members who interact significantly with patients on the unit, it is the patients' primary physicians who will generally be responsible for requesting consultation, for usefully assimilating the information provided, for adopting the consultant's suggestions, for assessing the usefulness of the process, and for deciding whether to ask for more consultations in the future (Popkin et al. 1983). Therefore, it is necessary to engage in some mutual reflection and dialogue about the prospective consultation process: With what attitudes about each other's specialties do the consultant and consultee approach the consultation relationship? What are their styles of practice (Hengeveld and Rooymans 1983)?

Attitude of the Primary Physician Toward Psychiatry

Inquire about the prospective consultees' previous experiences with, training and expertise in, and feelings about psychiatry. Do they think it is a valid discipline with a substantive data base and significant and specific treatment outcomes? Do they have reservations about your training, competence, gender, age, or other attributes pertaining to your role as future consultant? Make it clear you are prepared to accept frank statements, both positive and negative. It is better to know from the beginning what disappointments the consultees have suffered in the past than to work under a mysterious cloud of suspicion and distrust.

The following questions concerning the consultees' attitudes and expectations should be addressed:

- What, if anything, do the consultees hope to gain from the consultation relationship (Karasu et al. 1977)?
- What emotional and behavioral diagnostic and therapeutic dilemmas concern them?
- Do they find psychiatric illnesses and the patients who suffer from them distasteful and alien, challenging, or appealing?
- Do they want to know more about psychiatric issues so as to work more knowledgeably with patients, or do they hope that the consultant will take problems, and perhaps patients themselves, off their hands?
- Do they expect that the consultant will handle every problem with a psychoactive drug?

Attitude of the Psychiatric Consultant Toward the Consultee

Prospective consultants must ask analogous questions of themselves. We must introspectively examine our reactions to a consultee specialty, unit, and individual practice style, and individual consultee colleagues. We, too, have fears, hopes, and expectations based on our past experiences with the various medical, surgical, gynecologic, and pediatric specialties and subspecialties. Consultation is an interface at which medical approaches and styles meet. Not only does it inherently involve different specialties, but it often brings together a primary practitioner and a tertiary-care specialist, a hospital-based practitioner with one who is office-based, an academic or salaried practitioner with one who is in private practice. We all have feelings about our choices of practice and the others that we did not choose. Feelings that are acknowledged tend to interfere less with productive work.

It is difficult to make generalizations about feelings toward other specialties and practice patterns. Studies indicate that members of each specialty tend to have characteristic personality styles. Psychiatrists are likely to be intellectual and contemplative, while surgeons are action- or intervention-oriented. Just as other physicians sometimes wonder how anyone could choose to work with psychiatrically ill patients, psychiatrists may have little empathy for practitioners of trauma surgery or oncology. They may question the use of toxic chemotherapy or disfiguring surgery in patients with advanced malignancies, or the interventions of routine obstetric care, for example.

On the other hand, psychiatrists may also be consciously or unconsciously jealous about the lives they did not choose to lead. Many of us occasionally wish to enjoy the immediate gratification of a surgeon, who in a few hours or minutes removes an acutely inflamed appendix just before it ruptures, or reams out a clogged carotid artery in time to forestall a stroke. In any case, the consultant will have to understand and come to terms with the practices on the consultee service. This is almost never a problem in the long run: Once involved with a unit, the consultant will become identified with it and invested in alleviating the frustrations of colleagues and the suffering of patients.

Consultee Practice Patterns As They Relate to Consultation

Preparatory discussions with prospective consultees offer a valuable source of baseline information about their styles of practice as these styles affect the consultees' relationships with patients they will refer, and the working relationship with the consultant. For example, does the primary physician work with patients over many years, getting to know them, their families, and their typical responses to illness? Or do doctor and patient interact only around specific clinical situations, such as the need for surgery? Is contact limited to crises, in a consultation setting such as the emergency room?

Does the primary physician see the psychosocial needs of patients as an intrinsic part of illness and an appropriate focus of medical attention? Are consultation requests likely to be made emergently, or as a result of more extended contemplation and reflection in a diagnostically or therapeutically frustrating case? What is the usual style of doctor-patient interaction—authoritarian or collaborative, rushed or leisurely? The knowledge the consultant garners from these preparatory discussions will be greatly enriched by time, practice, and liaison activities. Such a discussion, in an atmosphere of flexibility and neutrality, can also inspire the new consultee to reflect about the implications of practice style, open a dialogue about it, and serve as a model for junior colleagues' professional behavior.

Using the information derived from the preliminary discussions, decide whether it will be necessary to negotiate a detailed structure for the consultation service. Is there sufficient latitude to allow for ad hoc arrangements? Or is the pace too fast and pressured? For example, will the consultee expect, and/or be available, to discuss cases before and after consultation? Consultant and consultee need to know how and when each can be reached. Fruitless paging and message leaving are sources of frustration and bad feelings.

Becoming Familiar With the Consultee Specialty

The fact that the psychiatric consultant is a physician is a vital fact of the consultation process. In an ongoing consultation relationship, it is both interesting and necessary to keep up with medical developments in the specialty to which one is consulting. Under optimal circumstances, one chooses a specialty in which one has an interest. Consultation is an opportunity to keep one's hand in another field, perhaps a field that captured one's interest in medical school but was relinquished in favor of psychiatry. Nearly any specialty becomes interesting once one becomes involved.

Core issues in the consultee area are psychiatric manifestations of disease processes, complications, and treatments, and the particular symptoms and concerns patients experience in the process of illness and treatment. Attendance at scientific functions and case conferences will broaden the knowledge base, keep it up to date, and demonstrate one's interest to consultees. Consultees and consultant will get to know one another in the scientific setting, and share ideas and curbstone consultations.

Becoming Familiar With the Institution

Learn about the schedules, rules, and patient population of the hospital and unit. Their relevance to consultation is apparent. The following issues should be addressed:

- When do doctors, nurses, and other staff make rounds? Are there separate work rounds and teaching rounds?
- What is the nurses' schedule? (When the shift is about to change, they are busy with reports.)
- What are the policies regarding numbers, relationships, and ages of visitors? Can someone stay overnight with a patient?
- Are there special rules for patients who are in intensive care, dying, or in labor? Are there different rules for private and clinic patients?
- Are there security issues: visitors who supply patients with substances of abuse and/or threaten the safety or possessions of patients? What are the resources for dealing with security needs?
- Is there a patient representative who mediates between patients and administration?
- Are there volunteers available to make social contact with patients, bring them recreational or personal materials, and/or perform personal services such as helping with shampooing, shaving, or makeup?
- Does the unit have educational materials on television or telephone to teach patients about diseases, treatments, examinations, and hospital procedures?

This information can enrich the content of consultation recommendations.

Teaching

Teaching is a doubly valuable means of access to a consultee service. It must be responsive to the needs, wishes, and limitations of the staff and institution. Often it is preferable to participate in an ongoing teaching or clinical exercise, rather than to impose another event on a crowded schedule and a harassed staff. There are situations in which a new conference, regular or occasional, is welcome. The support and attendance of the attending staff are crucial to the willing participation and respect of the house staff, who will know what time is best for the conference to be held. For nurses, a time around the change of shift may double the attendance.

Common psychiatric issues (anxiety, depression, somatization, sexual dysfunction), psychiatric concomitants of the consultee specialty, and discussions of current case and/or staff problems (by request only) are good topics. The format might be a brief discussion during work rounds, a case conference at attending rounds, a seminar, or a formal "grand rounds" lecture. The staff members who are responsible for planning regularly scheduled conferences are nearly always delighted to find a volunteer.

Find out who schedules teaching exercises on "your" consultee service. Physicians associate audiovisual aids with scientific accuracy. Handouts are appreciated and remind the participants of the consultant. Handouts may be bibliographies, outline summaries of the topic, salient papers from the literature, and/or key points of diagnosis, treatment, or referral. Handouts should always include the consultant's name and telephone number.

Working With a Known Service

The following are issues in the reorganization of existing psychiatric consultation services. Some of them apply to new services as well:

- Specify what services will now be offered, and at what hours.
- Distribute a call schedule. Make it clear what is to be done in the case of emergency and/or after-hours referrals.
- Delineate the division of clinical responsibility for referred patients between the primary physician and the consultant: Who will be expected to write orders? In most settings, the primary physician writes the orders, but in some institutions consultants provide direct care in their areas of expertise.
- How are consultations to be billed and paid for?
- Are consultations available to all patients, regardless of ability

to pay? If not, who will make the determination? Who will be responsible for the safety and well-being of patients financially ineligible for consultation services?

Resources for psychiatric inpatient and outpatient care are a frequent source of misunderstanding and frustration in psychiatric consultation work. Primary physicians are often unaware of the discriminatory nature of insurance coverage and are shocked to learn that the lack of coverage for psychiatric care may impede the transfer of patients who need psychiatric hospitalization. They may also be unaware, and annoyed, that many psychiatric inpatient units are limited in numbers of beds and types of patients who can be accommodated. A particularly difficult issue is the transfer or admission of medically ill patients. Some psychiatric facilities are not equipped or staffed to handle acute medical problems. These limitations contribute to tensions between psychiatry and other areas of medicine; the consultant must be prepared to discuss them openly and informatively, and address them constructively.

ROLE OF THE PSYCHIATRIST AS CONSULTANT

The question of professional identity is central to the function of a psychiatric consultant. The sometimes difficult distinctions between the roles of psychiatrists and other mental health professionals should be articulated for other primary-care physicians and consumers. Members of each discipline have particular expertise in one or more facets of mental health work, such as neuropsychological testing or the use of community resources, both of which are particularly valuable in work with general hospital patients. Workers of many disciplines may have psychotherapeutic skills and interests: psychoanalysis, psychodynamic psychotherapy, behavioral techniques, family and group therapy, crisis intervention, supportive therapy.

Unique to psychiatrists is the medical training that prepares us to assess the interactions between physical and emotional manifestations of so-called "somatic" and "functional" psychiatric illnesses and to treat patients with the whole spectrum of therapies, including manipulation of medications prescribed for other conditions, psychoactive drugs, electroconvulsive therapy (ECT) and other somatic therapies, and psychiatric hospitalization. These qualifications, which are sometimes unclear to nonpsychiatric physicians, are the reason why final responsibility for the safety and care of psychiatrically ill patients rests most safely, clinically and legally, with psychiatric physicians.

REFERENCES

Abel GG, Rouleau J-L, Coyne BJ: Behavioral medicine strategies in medical patients, in Principles of Medical Psychiatry. Edited by Stoudemire MD, Fogel BS. Orlando, FL, Grune & Stratton, 1987, pp 329–345

Adler G: Helplessness in the helpers. Br J Med Psychol 45:315–326, 1972

Engel GL: The need for a new medical model. Science 196:129–136, 1977

Fogel BS, Faust D: Neurologic assessment, neurodiagnostic tests, and neuropsychology in medical psychiatry, in Principles of Medical Psychiatry. Edited by Stoudemire MD, Fogel BS. Orlando, FL, Grune and Stratton, 1987, pp 37–77

Hawkins DR: The gap between the psychiatrist and other physicians. Psychosom Med 24:1–5, 1962

Hengeveld NW, Rooymans HGM: The relevance of a staff-oriented approach in consultation psychiatry: a preliminary study. Gen Hosp Psychiatry 5:259–264, 1983

Karasu TB, Plutchnik R, Conte H, et al: What do physicians want from a psychiatric consultation service? Compr Psychiatry 18:73–81, 1977

Lipowski ZJ: Review of consultation psychiatry and psychosomatic medicine. I. General principles. Psychosom Med 29:153–171, 1967

Lipowski ZJ: Consultation-liaison psychiatry: an overview. Am J Psychiatry 131:623–630, 1974

Mohl PC: The liaison psychiatrist: social role and status. Psychosomatics 20:19–23, 1977

Mohl PC: Working with the nursing staff, in Manual of Psychiatric Consultation and Emergency Care. Edited by Guggenheim FG, Weiner MF. New York, Jason Aronson, 1984, pp 255–263

O'Connor S, Bilodeau CB: The psychiatric nurse clinical specialist in liaison psychiatry, in Massachusetts General Hospital Handbook of General Hospital Psychiatry, 2nd Edition. Edited by Hackett TP, Cassem NH. Littleton, MA, PSG Publishing, 1987, pp 572–590

Popkin MK, Mackenzie TB, Callies AL: Consultation-liaison outcome evaluation system. I. Consultant-consultee interaction. Arch Gen Psychiatry 40:215–219, 1983

Schwab J: Handbook of Psychiatric Consultation. New York, Appleton-Century-Crofts, 1968

3

Initiating the Consultation

In this chapter, we detail the specific mechanisms by which psychiatric consultation is requested and set in motion. This intake process is the interface between the consultation seeker and the consultation provider. The content, workability, and reliability of these mechanisms often determine whether a consultation will actually take place, how smoothly it will begin, and whether and/or how future consultations will be contemplated by the primary care provider (Gobar et al. 1987).

The potential consultant must always bear in mind the fact that psychiatric consultation may be seen as optional in the medical care of the patient. On the other hand, a call for psychiatric consultation is often made when the consultee perceives the situation to be an emergency, as when the patient threatens violence against himself or herself, or against others (Fulop and Strain 1986), refuses important medical procedures (Himmelhoch et al. 1970), or attempts to leave the hospital prematurely (Colon et al. 1988). In the busy world of the general hospital and its staff, uncertainty about whom to call, a telephone number not immediately at hand, an unanswered telephone, or any other obstacle, may result in failure to make (or delay in making) the contact, thus impeding the work of primary physician and consultant and the care of the patient (Cassem and Hackett 1971). Therefore, we explain how to make the intake procedure as clear, easy, and reliable as possible.

PREARRANGEMENTS

As discussed below, the potential consultant will meet with the heads and staffs of clinical services in advance to discuss in depth what consultation services are desired and can be provided, and how the procedure might best operate to meet the specific circumstances and needs of the unit. At the time of these discussions, leave your card or name and pager/telephone number with each of the staff members concerned, and at the nursing station, clinic desk, or other central locations where clinical-care decisions are made and arranged. This reminder gives information about how to reach you for further discussion while the details of the consultation arrangement are being formulated.

THE CONSULTATION INFORMATION CARD

After considering the setup of the unit and your particular practice style, distribute printed information about the new consultation service. The composition of this printed information must balance completeness against brevity. Label the document clearly: for example, "Psychiatric Consultation Service." Indicate that the document is to be posted by the telephone of each nursing station or wherever other such information is displayed.

List the name of the psychiatrist—you or your designee—who will respond to consultation requests. Make it clear whether the initial consultant will be a psychiatric resident or an attending psychiatrist; if he or she is a member of the house staff, who is the responsible attending psychiatrist? If there is to be a system of rotation or frequent changes of psychiatric personnel, decide whether to include the roster or simply offer a central number. Individual names are more appealing; it is always most comfortable to know whom one is calling. On the other hand, a complex or out-of-date schedule is confusing, misleading, and possibly unnecessary. Will the consultees care who the specific consultant is?

Having made these decisions during the prearrangement period, update your document using the results of your ongoing clinical consultation experience. When the contact psychiatrists are members of the house staff, and/or when there are a number of them, you may want to list the name and number of the attending psychiatrist who is director of the service and state that this psychiatrist may be contacted whenever there is doubt about how to proceed, a problem, difficulty reaching the designated consultant, a question, or dissatisfaction concerning psychiatric consultation. For a large hospital consultation service, you may want to develop both a large master information sheet and cards for each clinical service, specifying the routes to particular consultants, in order to provide individualized service and simplify access.

Make it clear at what hours specific consultants are to be contacted and telephone or pager numbers are to be used. Try to simplify the system rather than the information card. The primary care provider can request a psychiatric consultation without knowing which psychiatrist will respond, but not without knowing what number to call. If he or she finds it necessary to look up the general number of the psychiatry department, the result may be an angry call to the chairperson. And if an attempt to get through fails, other pressing issues in patient care may take priority (Krakowski 1975). By the time the thought recurs, the patient's condition may have deteriorated or the patient may have been discharged from the hospital.

In some hospitals, there is a "drop box" system. Written requests for consultation can be deposited in a mail box, either in the psychiatry department or in a central location used for consultation requests to other departments. If a box is used, deposits must be picked up reliably and often, by a clearly designated member of the professional or support staff, and provision made for monitoring or substitute arrangements for emergencies and night, weekend, and holiday coverage.

We refer to the printed information as a "card" because it should be as durable, compact, formal, and noticeable as possible. Your announcement will vie for attention—and physical space—with the many others posted in every care station. Develop a format that highlights the most important and frequently needed information. Cards are available in bright colors and can be small enough to fit into a lab-coat pocket. Keep the information on the card absolutely current, and use every opportunity to distribute updated versions, not only to care stations but to individual staff members. These updated cards are a welcome and practical hand-out at lectures and rounds.

THE CONSULTEE

A crucial factor in the preliminary arrangements is the decision as to who will have the responsibility for and privilege of calling a psychiatric consultant in on a case. Most commonly, this is the primary physician. Medical tradition, as well as many third-party payers, requires that only a physician be empowered to request a consultation from another physician. The Joint Commission on Accreditation of Hospitals requires that a psychiatrist be called whenever a patient is noted to experience suicidal ideation and whenever a patient's care necessitates interventions beyond the expertise of the primary physician (JCAH 1965). In fact, the consultation is conceptualized or defined as observations and recommendations offered to the patient's doctor (Lipowski 1974).

The primary physician, or hospital physician of record, has clinical and legal responsibility for the patient and for all orders issued pursuant to the patient's care. In some hospitals, only orders written or countersigned by the attending physician are valid, while in others, concurrent care providers and house staff can also enter orders in the chart. In still others, to prevent contradictory or confusing orders issuing from a multiplicity of care providers, and to utilize the physician most often physically present in the hospital, only the intern enters orders.

When only the physician writes the orders, hospitals or treatment teams may agree that others may initiate a consultation. The consultant needs to be thoroughly conversant with the system in force on the consultee unit and to clearly designate from whom requests will be entertained.

For a variety of reasons, persons other than the physician of record may recognize and voice the need for psychiatric consultation. House and nursing staff generally spend more time at the inpatient bedside than attending staff. They often detect subtle mood and mental status changes not apparent in brief contacts during attending rounds. Social workers are familiar with the effects of particular illnesses and situations on patients and families and can identify those at particular risk. Physical and occupational therapists often work intensely with patients and recognize mental deterioration.

Patients and members of their families occasionally ask for a psychiatric consultation because of painful emotional symptoms, previous successful psychiatric contacts, problematic behaviors, or a history of and/or current known major psychiatric illness. Once a workable system of consultation is in place, the primary physician is usually more than willing to arrange for a psychiatrist to see the patient (Brown and Cooper 1987).

Hospital mental health professionals other than psychiatrists—chaplain counselors, social workers, and psychologists—may have seen a patient and identified a need for psychiatric referral. Psychologists generally see patients in response to specific requests from the service, while on some units chaplains and social workers screen either all patients or those with designated risk factors, those belonging to certain religious groups, those requesting service, or those presenting specific psychosocial problems ranging from emotional symptoms to discharge planning.

CALLING MECHANISMS

Since the mechanisms of consultation are so critical to its success, review not only the acceptable sources of consultation requests but also precisely who will make the calls to set these requests in motion. Will it be the attending physician, the resident, the nurse, or the ward clerk?

Who receives the call? This may be a previously specified consultant—either a psychiatrist who is on the staff and in private practice, a salaried staff member of a private institution, or a member of the faculty or house staff of a teaching hospital. Will the number offered the consultee service provide access to the psychiatrist or the psychiatrist's secretary or answering service? These call recipients must be fully prepared to make the caller feel that the call is welcome, that its purpose is understood, and that the message will be respected and efficiently conveyed. A specific reference to the time the consultant is next expected to return or pick up messages is reassuring to the caller.

Call Coverage

When a call must be placed to a consultation service rather than a specific consultant, it is even more important to assure the caller that the request will be expeditiously handled. Psychiatrists must be seen to be available and responsive when they are needed (Schwab 1968). Ideally, the consultation service has enough volume to justify the employment of its own coordinator who takes calls, assigns cases, and keeps track of completed consultations, follow-ups, dispositions, and overall statistics. Someone knowledgeable and responsible must answer the consultation number, at least during all normal working hours, and, of course, advance provision will have been made for emergency requests at any hour.

In our experience, the absence of the usual coordinator or secretary has been the occasion for serious problems in the communication of requests for consultation and the provision of care, resulting in considerable confusion, consternation, complaints, accusations, and disillusionment by consultees. The inevitable breaks for vacations, illness, and even lunch and errands must be covered and trouble anticipated. Consultants on call have to check frequently for messages. The covering secretarial staff member must be educated as to the workings, purpose, and importance of the consultation mechanism. Performance must be monitored, mishaps investigated and explained, and effectiveness appreciated and acknowledged.

Another problematic interface is the relaying of requests and cases from off-hour psychiatrists covering the consultation service to the regular consultation staff. The consultees tend to see the psychiatry department or service as a unity. Once psychiatric contact has been initiated, they expect ongoing psychiatric care and follow-up, and do not tend to call in a formal request even when there is a mechanism for doing so. Therefore, any member of the psychiatry staff who sees a general hospital patient in consultation must remain responsible for the psychiatric care of that patient until the case has been officially presented to, and care undertaken by, the consultation service or an individual consultant.

Paging Systems. Paging systems, or "beepers," are an

increasingly common and useful route for requests for consultation. They enable a primary-care practitioner to reach a specific consultant without the intervention of an intermediary. They enable consultants to be available on a 24-hour basis, or on any prearranged, consistent, and workable basis, without sitting by a telephone or checking constantly for messages. There are several common problems, however. Pagers seem to be more vulnerable to malfunction than telephones. Systems often necessitate dialing in a change of location as the consultant moves within and without the hospital, and this step can easily be forgotten, leading to unanswered pages.

The pager offers an illusion of constant availability that must be either met or addressed. What will happen when you are conducting a session with a patient, stuck in traffic or in another situation without a phone available, or in a crowded outside setting where there is a long wait for the phone? Decide, and make clear to consultees, beforehand how these situations will be handled. Should you sign out to someone more available? Should the consultee seek someone else after a certain period of time has elapsed?

Triage. Another issue in coverage is triage. Settle on a time frame within which routine, urgent, and emergency consultations will be seen, and give each a formal designation so that both caller and call receiver are clear as to which is being requested. Educating potential consultees about the criteria for each of these designations is a separate part of the psychiatrist's task. In many settings, a specific psychiatrist cannot promise to see a patient immediately even during normal working hours. Emergency care is provided by house staff, for example, by the resident on call for the emergency room, or under a rotating call system.

It is vitally important that every call be answered as quickly as possible. A consultation is requested because the primary team is unsure about the patient's condition and care. Although they may attempt to perform their own triage, their psychiatric sophistication is, by definition, insufficient to address the patient's problem. Delaying the response to the initial call only increases their anxiety. Talk to a member of the team who knows the patient's situation and ask whatever you need to know (see below) to determine the urgency of the need for your presence (Popkin and Mackenzie 1984).

Inform the caller as to when the patient will be seen. A commonly used rule of thumb is that routine consultations are accomplished within 24 working hours, urgent ones within a few hours, and emergent ones as soon as humanly possible. The person who answers the call should also be prepared to advise the caller on emergency interventions for patients who present an immediate danger to themselves or others. Primary physicians and others involved in care, once they are aware of inpatient consultation availability, often call for advice about outpatients as well. They may, for example, be advised to take the patient to the emergency room, call the police, and/or see that someone is with the patient at all times.

Sometimes the intake process also involves a differentiation among patients who belong to various care systems. Health maintenance and other relatively new care systems may have designated consultants on their own staffs. The psychiatric consultant may respond to a request for service and complete the workup before discovering that the patient belongs to such a plan and that the completed consultation will be neither utilized nor reimbursed. In other cases, the patient may have an ongoing therapeutic relationship with a psychiatrist who has not been informed of the patient's admission to the hospital but who is available and competent to follow the case through the medical illness.

At the same time, the members of the psychiatric consultation service may want to be at least informed about, if not more active in the care of, all patients with psychiatric problems in the medical units they serve. The consultee service often does not differentiate among mental health–care providers, and will attribute any such care provided to the psychiatry department. It not uncommonly happens, especially when the mental health–care provider is not a physician, that the psychiatric consultant or service is called when the patient's condition deteriorates or when an emergency, difficult decision, or disposition problem arises.

INFORMATION TO REQUEST

Rationale

The decision about what information to elicit from the caller requesting psychiatric consultation for a patient involves the same weighing of completeness against brevity as do so many other issues in the consultation process. On one hand, we do not want to encumber the request, or deter the caller, with an exhaustive list of questions. When the caller is a clerk or other staff member who does not know the patient, and the consultant plans to call the responsible physician and/or appear on the hospital unit immediately, you may require only enough information to locate and identify the patient.

On the other hand, preliminary information can help focus the consultant's thoughts in advance and even help him or her begin to frame realistic expectations about what the consultation may accomplish. If the service plans to discharge the patient that day or the next, for example, it becomes less likely that a full psychiatric workup can be completed and that the consultant can achieve sufficient rapport with the patient to increase the likelihood of compliance with a referral for inpatient or outpatient psychiatric care. The consultant may want to review, mentally or in a personal or hospital library, the characteristic problems of patients with the medical illness of the referred patient, or those of patients with the same presenting issues or in the same demographic group.

Specific pieces of information also help the consultant locate the consultee for an important preliminary contact (see Chapter 4), ensure that the consultee is entitled to request consultation, and weed out cases whose consultation needs are to be served by another source (within or without a health maintenance organization [HMO], for example). When, as is optional, potential consultees and consultants have mutually worked out beforehand what questions will be asked when the call is made, the need to gather the data helps the consultee formulate the situation and the reasons for and goals of the consultation.

Thinking constructively about these questions can even shape the primary physician's behavior toward more effective collaboration with the consultation service. For example, we routinely encourage medical services to request consultation as early as possible in the patient's course. A consultation on a patient about to be discharged, or requested because a patient whose physical workup was either negative or prognostically dire, is limited from the beginning by time constraints and/or the hostile or distracted attitude of the patient. A potential consultee thoroughly familiar with the agreement that the patient's dates of admission and probable discharge will be requested when a consultation is called in is probably more likely to call early enough to allow time for effective psychiatric evaluation and treatment planning.

Specific Pieces of Information

The consultee will need the name and geographic location of the patient. Careful spelling, a hospital patient or unit number, and a bed number will minimize the chance of mistaken identity. Other highly useful pieces of information about the patient are age, sex, date of admission, reason for admission, medical diagnosis, and medical condition.

What is the reason for psychiatric referral? You might want to include a question about what specific behavior of the patient precipitated the request for consultation. The reason alone may mislead the consultant about the urgency of the clinical situation. For example, a complaint of "suicidal" may be precipitated by the refusal of the patient to sign consent for a procedure deemed crucial by the service. The complaint "rule out depression" may be precipitated by the patient's expression of a wish to die. "Bizarre behavior" can indicate actions that threaten the safety of patient or staff.

Also useful are the names and telephone or pager numbers of the attending physician, primary-care nurse, if any, intern, and resident. If possible, find out whose idea it was to ask for the consultation. This person is likely to be the most motivated and knowledgeable about the problem for which consultation is sought.

Is the consultation urgent or emergent? Is the request for a full workup or for a limited kind of information such as medication dosage or the name of an appropriate outpatient psychiatrist in

the community? The approach to these requests for limited consultation, and to dealing with the problem identified by the consultee as the reason for consultation in general, is discussed in
subsequent chapters of this manual.

RECORDING AND CONVEYING THE INFORMATION

On one-person or small consultation services, and where calls are
placed directly to the consultant, the latter may simply elicit and
jot down the information during the call. But on services where a
secretary or coordinator actually receives the requests, or where
more careful record keeping is desired, a request form should be
prepared. Instruct everyone who answers the consultation phone
in the proper completion of the form. Do not expect a non-
psychiatrist to remember or appreciate the array of information
important to the consultant.

The same form or an adjunct form may also address needs
beyond the initial contact. Register the date and time of consultation, the amount of time spent, persons contacted, and dates,
times, and durations of additional diagnostic visits and activities
(discussions with outside or past therapists, family meetings,
staff conferences) carried out to further the evaluation and care of
the patient. The highlights of the consultation conclusions are
often noted. These include (a) the psychiatric diagnosis, (b) evalu-
ative procedures (e.g., psychological testing, computed axial
tomography [CAT] scan, electroencephalographic neurological
consultation) and specific treatments (e.g., drugs and dosages,
psychotherapy with a particular mental health–care provider,
inpatient substance abuse program) recommended, (c) actual disposition, and (d) outcome to date.

Such forms can be developed and used for many different purposes to suit the needs of the individual consultation arrangement. They facilitate record keeping that is designed to document
time and activities invested in patient care. These forms can then
support needs ranging from billing to the hiring of additional
psychiatric staff. They enable the service to see how it is spending
its time and facilitate the consideration and periodic reconsideration of priorities, needs, problems, and effectiveness.

Consultation request forms can fairly easily be prepared to be
suitable for computerized processing and record keeping. This is

extremely useful for the service documentation and billing just discussed, and for teaching, improved care, and research as well. An appropriate computer program (some are commercially available) enables the service director, attending psychiatrist, and resident to track how many consultations a trainee has undertaken, and the array of demographic characteristics and medical and psychiatric diagnoses of the patients involved (Hale and De L'Aune 1983). Provisions can be made during training to modify the consultation case load or mix of a resident to offer experience with a wide array of clinical cases.

Careful or computerized record keeping can also focus teaching and hiring needs. If there is a large or increasing load of geriatric patients, or of those with a particular kind of diagnosis, teaching conferences can address the related issues, and subspecialty staff can be trained or hired. Easily traced trends in referring patterns from various medical units may also reflect the effectiveness or ineffectiveness of liaison efforts. These kinds of information have also been used for formal research. A multicenter collaborative effort has been active for some time (Hammer et al. 1985).

Conclusions

Attention to the details of the referral process, examined in this chapter, is crucial to the success of psychiatric consultation. Simplicity, accessibility, clarity, the exchange of information, and record keeping require painstaking thought, planning, and monitoring. But they also demonstrate commitment, enhance the likelihood of requests for consultation, and improve patient care, psychiatric training, and research into vital psychosomatic and care-provision issues.

References

Brown A, Cooper AF: The impact of a liaison psychiatry service on patterns of referral in a general hospital. Br J Psychiatry 150:83–87, 1987

Cassem NH, Hackett TP: Psychiatric consultation in a coronary care unit. Ann Intern Med 75:9–14, 1971

Colon EA, Popkin M, Callies A: Emergency psychiatric consultation to medical-surgical services. Psychosomatics 29:3–10, 1988

Fulop G, Strain JJ: Psychiatric emergencies in the general hospital. Gen Hosp Psychiatry 8:425–431, 1986

Gobar AH, Collins JL, Mathura CB: Why doctors do and don't call psychiatry. JAMA 79:505–508, 1987

Hale MS, De L'Aune W: Microcomputer use on a consultation-liaison service. Psychosomatics 25:1003–1015, 1983

Hammer JS, Hammond D, Strain JJ, et al: Microcomputers and consultation psychiatry in the general hospital. Gen Hosp Psychiatry 7:119–124, 1985

Himmelhoch JM, Davies RK, Tucker GJ, et al: Butting heads: patients who refuse necessary procedures. Int J Psychiatry Med 1:241–249, 1970

Joint Commission on Accreditation of Hospitals: Report of the Joint Commission. Chicago, IL, Joint Commission on the Accreditation of Hospitals, 1965

Krakowski AJ: Psychiatric consultation in the general hospital: an exploration of resistances. Diseases of the Nervous System 36:242–244, 1975

Lipowski ZJ: Consultation-liaison psychiatry: an overview. Am J Psychiatry 131:623–630, 1974

Popkin MK, Mackenzie TB: Communicating with the referring physician, in Manual of Psychiatric Consultation and Emergency Care. Edited by Guggenheim FG, Weiner MF. New York, Jason Aronson, 1984, pp 115–123

Schwab J: Handbook of Psychiatric Consultation. New York, Appleton-Century-Crofts, 1968

4

Contacting the Referring Service

Underscoring the psychiatric consultation as an interaction between two medical experts is the need to begin every consultation by contacting the primary or referring physician (Lipowski 1967). This need is pertinent regardless of the institutional structure within which the consultation takes place (Glazer and Astrachan 1978–1979). There are issues of timing, of identifying the appropriate doctor(s) or other staff members to see or call, of deciding what information to seek, and of setting up the contract for the initial consultation.

This step in the consultation may seem superfluous. If a consultation has been requested and will be performed, why not proceed directly to the patient's bedside and get to work? Often it is difficult to reach the referring physician, who may commute between offices and institutions, attend meetings, and/or be involved in surgical or other procedures that cannot be interrupted. And you, the consultant, may be difficult to reach when a call is returned; you too commute, attend meetings, and engage in therapeutic procedures that ought not be disturbed. However, the failure to accomplish this first step can obscure and undermine the goals and process of the entire consultation. Without this step, the consultant may be operating at cross purposes with the consultee or be deprived of information vital to the diagnosis or therapeutic recommendations.

TIMING

The best time to call the referring physician is immediately. A consultation is requested because the consultee is not an expert in psychiatry and has recognized a need for specialized assistance. In addition, if the consultation has been requested through one or more intermediaries (ward clerks, secretaries, social workers), it is always possible that there has been some misunderstanding as to the urgency of the need for psychiatric intervention, or the time when it will be initiated. Therefore, it is prudent to make one's own judgment, as quickly as possible, as to the urgency of the need for consultation, and to make sure that one's schedule for the consultation agrees, or is brought into agreement, with the expectations of the consultee.

The same logic applies when the need for a consultation has been mentioned—in conversation or at rounds, for example—but no formal request has been received. It is noteworthy how, despite repeated reminders about the mechanism for requesting consultations, primary providers may still assume that a consultation will be performed simply because they have thought about it. Sometimes there is only a mention in the chart that the possibility is being considered, without any communication at all to the psychiatrists responsible for consultation. Yet the primary service becomes irate that the patient has not been evaluated and cared for, or proceeds, without noticing, to treat and discharge the patient without the indicated psychiatric intervention.

One may not wish, or in some settings be able, to proceed without a formal request. In these cases, it is often advisable to pursue the involved physician and clarify the situation. However, when it is clear that there is a wish for a consultation, with no disagreement among the staff, some consultants see the patient and enter a consultation note in the chart, with the written request form to be signed afterward by the designated member of the primary-care team. An unrequested and undesired intervention could cause trouble; the primary physician and patient would correctly view this as an intrusion.

We have not had significant problems with such situations. It is preferable to err on the side of providing timely service to patients and physicians in need. When there is good reason to think that a consultation is desired, and the primary or referring physician cannot be contacted, proceed at least far enough with the consultation to ascertain that there is no psychiatric emergency. Insisting on formalities may at times deprive patients of clinically important assessment and treatment.

WHOM TO CONTACT

The aims of the contact (see below) dictate the persons to be called or seen. The consultant needs to speak to the physician in charge of the patient, the person who decided there was need for consultation, and the staff member who knows most about the patient's current condition (Meyer and Mendelson 1961). Ideally, these are one and the same individual. Sometimes, however, they are three different persons, and only persistent tracking enables the consultant to identify and locate each one.

In fact, it may not be immediately clear just who is the responsible physician. Consulting psychiatrists, who are not generally part of the day-to-day workings of the general hospital unit, may not be aware of the policies and realities with reference to responsibility and the writing of orders. Hospital accreditation and third-party-payer requirements dictate that an attending staff physician be responsible for each patient. In practice, the implementation of this rule ranges from hands-on, daily care to periodic signing of charts.

The name the consultant is likely to have is that of the person who officially requested that the patient be seen. Begin by calling that person. If he or she is both knowledgeable and available, the preliminary business can be transacted. If he or she says, "I was just told to call," "I don't know why they want psychiatry to see this patient," "I'm just covering the service," etc., it will be necessary to ask who would know why the request has been made, and who is responsible for the patient.

Even in a setting where members of the house staff have nearly total responsibility for, and wide latitude in, patient care, it is almost always useful, or even vital, to contact the attending physician. This contact conveys respect for his or her role and responsibility. The attending physician may be opposed to the idea and agree only after discussion with the consultant. The attending physician may have suggested the consultation. This call may elicit useful information, since the attending physician has more experience and sophistication in a particular clinical area than a member of the junior house staff. It also establishes or confirms a link with a staff member who will remain on, or repeatedly rotate through, the service for years, caring for patients, teaching young physicians, and setting a tone for the relationship with psychiatry (Borus and Casserly 1979). In a private-practice setting, the private attending physician generally expects to be kept informed about all developments affecting the patient and is a continuing source of referrals for the psychiatrist (Popkin and Mackenzie 1984).

On occasion, no physician responsible for the patient can be reached right away. Recourse may then be made to any staff member, especially if the request for consultation conveys any sense of urgency. If the request originated with someone other than the primary physician, both this person and the physician may be called.

INFORMATION SOUGHT

Nature of the Clinical Problem[1]

"Medical" Aspects.   First of all, inquire as to the patient's medical diagnosis and current condition. Much information never reaches the chart, and important elements of the physician's thinking can be captured only in person-to-person contact. A brief summary of the differential diagnosis can bring the psychiatrist up to date on the scientific knowledge in a subspecialty area as it pertains to the patient, and focus the psychiatric evaluation on the particular items of information that would be of use.

The contact also reveals nuances in the specifics of the medical workup and management or in the attitudes of the staff who are caring for the patient. The doctor may betray annoyance, bewilderment, hopelessness, and/or like or dislike for the patient (Groves 1978). Troublesome and/or worrisome behaviors of the

---

[1]The words "medical" and "psychiatric" are introduced in quotation marks in this section because these aspects of the clinical situation are, of course, inseparable facets of the same psychobiological condition. They are considered separately here because our medical colleagues, and society at large, think in terms of these concepts. In order to communicate, we have to be able to begin in these common frames of reference and then educate consultees about inherent interrelationships (Engel 1977).

patient or relatives with respect to medical conditions and compliance may be mentioned (Strain 1978). These will shed light both on the reason the primary physician is asking for help and on the condition of the patient and the psychosocial surround (Schiff and Pilot 1959). A common example is a situation in which the patient has been admitted after days of frequent calls to the physician and/or visits to the emergency service or office. The real reason for admission is the patient's personality style, psychosocial crisis, or response to medically trivial symptoms. The primary physician can also describe management that was attempted in the outpatient setting but not entered in the hospital chart.

Medical and psychosocial questions raised by the consultant not only elicit useful information but inform the primary physician about issues to be considered. The consultant can help him or her to structure observations and thoughts so as to clarify the question asked of the consultant, and the diagnosis and management of the patient in general. Specifics of the mental status examination are a very common example. After describing the patient's agitation and disorientation or memory loss, the referring physician may realize that the patient is delirious or demented.

The information about the patient's current medical condition is often a useful clue to the reason for the change in the patient's mood and/or behavior that occasioned the request for consultation. For example, the staff realizes, but does not voice, the fact that a patient has not responded favorably to the most rigorous and sophisticated treatment regimen available. They know that the patient is deteriorating and will not recover. The patient is not told this, but quickly senses it from the demeanor and communications of staff and family. Because no overt communication of the adverse prognosis has been made to the patient, no one can understand why the patient withdraws, ceases to comply or cooperate, seems resentful, or appears depressed (Konior and Levine 1975).

Another example is the case of the compliant and appreciative patient who has fought a brave battle with a severe disease and won the hearts of the medical team. When all the routes of aggressive, curative treatment are exhausted, and death appears inevitable, psychiatric consultation is requested in an effort to offer the patient one last humane and human resource. We arrive at the bedside to "rule out depression" and are bewildered to find a moribund patient who may even be completely unable to speak.

When the referring physician has taken care of the patient over time, the consultant can also use the initial contact to ask about medications and other treatments prescribed in the past. There may be correlations between discontinuations or dosages and variations in the problem for which consultation is sought. Perhaps the patient has a tendency to overuse benzodiazepines and is withdrawing from these agents, or was recently started on an antihypertensive agent associated with a significant incidence of depression.

Finally, it is often useful to know how the patient's general health has been over the years, and what has been his or her level of functioning in family, social, and work roles. Knowing that the patient was a vivacious, active, energetic person who was seldom ill, or, conversely, a chronically debilitated and weak invalid, puts the impressions obtained in the ensuing interview in a diagnostically and therapeutically important perspective. The temporal course of signs and symptoms is an essential component of differential diagnosis. For example, is the patient's current anxiety part of a lifelong pattern (Kahana and Bibring 1964), a frequent response to stress, or an unprecedented reaction? Often this history is also the best indicator of prognosis.

The questions raised by the consultant must be focused so as to be relevant to the consultee. They must fit within the time frame available for the initial contact. The first contact is not always the best time to engage in a detailed discussion of the entire case. We cannot interrupt a surgeon in the middle of a critical procedure. Psychiatrists vary widely in their approaches. As with all professional behaviors, one should get to know one's own strengths, weaknesses, and style. Some of us are too modest about the importance of our contributions, and overly concerned about taking up the time of the referring physician, patient, family, and staff. These are the same individuals who, unlike most physicians in other specialties, are loathe to delay the departure of a patient for a routine test, when, in fact, a special trip has been made to perform the consultation, or to ask the nurse whether the patient's bath might be postponed. Others may confidently or counterphobically assert themselves in an initial contact in such a way as to overwhelm or put off the consultee. These attitudes and behaviors are manifestations of ethnic background, values, and educational bias, as well as transference and countertransference. We might perceive the primary service as parental, or ourselves as saviors of a psychologically neglected patient. Variations in style are inevitable and even valuable so long as they do not interfere with professional relationships.

"Psychiatric" Aspects. As just mentioned, the referring physician may have a wealth of more or less explicit, organized, and applied information derived from clinical experience with the patient. There are three extremely valuable kinds of data to be sought in the initial contact: (1) baseline and/or changes in mental status; (2) baseline and/or changes in general functioning, responses to illness, personality style, family relationships, and relationships with physicians; and (3) past psychiatric history. Sometimes the amount of data is disappointing despite years of contact; nevertheless, the primary-care practitioner may be able to organize long-standing observations under the stimulus of focused questions, may remember and communicate other items after the conversation, and will also learn what to note in the future.

Mental status. Baseline mental status, including not only cognitive but also affective and behavioral factors, can be a crucial factor in both diagnosis and management. Each disease process has a characteristic curve of evolution. The consultant makes an observation at one point in time. Information supplied by the primary care provider can supply previous points on the curve. Later in the consultation process, when disposition is being considered, it will also be necessary to correlate the current mental status with the patient's ability to function in a given setting. Previous mental status and function are vital reference points.

Obviously, one needs to inquire first just how long the referring physician has known and cared for the patient. If the current consultee is new to the case, can anyone identify a professional care provider who has had previous contact? Try to get a sense of what the relationship entailed so that you can assess the probable accuracy of the information you receive, the likelihood that other data, if needed, may be available from the same source, and the usefulness of the relationship as a management and emotional resource for the patient (Balint 1957).

What is the primary physician's general sense of the patient's baseline and previous mental status, and his or her sense of what changes have occurred? It may be that continuing work with the patient has caused deficits to be taken for granted. Some specific questions may be helpful:

- Did the patient ever seem confused or disoriented? Were there episodes of wandering or other problematic behavior complained of by the patient or relatives?
- Could the patient manage complex therapeutic regimens? give an accurate history of the development of symptoms and the response to interventions? exhibit good judgment in making health-related decisions?

General function. The following questions concerning baseline general function may be helpful:

- What is the patient's educational background and previous level of intellectual function? What was the level of the patient's functioning in general? Has he or she always been a passive invalid, or a seeming victim of a succession of crises and tragedies? Or is the patient a person who has mastered many difficulties successfully, taken charge of most situations, taken care of others?
- What is the work history?
- What sort of a person has the patient been—in general personality style, in relation to significant others, and as a patient in relation to care providers? What helpful lessons has the primary physician gleaned from experience with this patient? For example, are frequent visits to the bedside required, or does the patient prefer to be left alone as much as possible? How has the patient handled previous illnesses and hospitalizations (Strain 1975)? Perhaps the current storm the patient has created is a typical one for him or her, and one that always resolves spontaneously. Perhaps the patient behaves in a certain way until important family members are mobilized. Does the

patient tend to be deeply skeptical about medical advice, or almost overly trusting?

Psychiatric history.

- What is known about the patient's psychiatric history proper? Did the patient complain of, or manifest, mood swings or extended periods of depressive and/or manic signs and symptoms? Were there bizarre behaviors and/or frank delusions or hallucinations suggestive of a thought disorder? The referring or primary physician may also have access to information about psychiatric events in the patient's family. Because of the past uncertainty and stigma of psychiatric illness, past episodes of psychosis or depression may only be known as "nervous breakdowns," or even as periods of time when the patient or near relative unaccountably withdrew from ordinary activities.
- Does the physician know who else might be knowledgeable and available to offer the consultant other information? Perhaps the physician can remember what mental health professional, clinic, or hospital treated the patient or what pharmacologic agents were used.

The Precipitant for Calling the Consultation

Very often, the stated reason for the consultation does not convey the proximate reason(s) the request was actually made (Schiff and Pilot 1959). Knowing the dynamics of the situation is crucial to focus, diagnosis, and management. Although the consultant is not the consultee's doctor, there are significant analogies between the doctor-patient encounter and the consultation. Knowing what a patient thinks is wrong, and what made him or her finally or actually call for an appointment, is a pivotal issue in every workup. The answers to these questions convey helpful diagnostic information. For example, the patient may have had a chief complaint of nonspecific, subacute abdominal pain, while the reason for the precipitant visit is hematemesis—an urgent medical problem. The patient may complain of headache but be privately convinced that the reason is the same sort of hypertension that led to a stroke in a parent. The patient is not likely to follow recommendations that do not address the underlying concerns for which medical care was sought. Those concerns must be refuted or gratified.

Similarly, a consultee may ask us to "rule out depression" when the patient is nagging, noncompliant, or despondent over what seems to be or is a dire prognosis. The consultee may expect a simple recommendation for a tricyclic antidepressant. Unless the consultant is prepared simply to fulfill this expectation, and not to address the underlying problem in the patient-care system, it will be necessary to determine what is really and acutely bothering the consultee.

If the precipitant for the consultation request was a call from a relative of the patient, that relationship will have to be dealt with. If the patient's chronic behavior annoys the primary physician, it will be necessary to offer recommendations for changing that behavior or the response to it. If the precipitant was an episode during which the patient wandered around the hospital unit and disturbed other patients and staff, recommendations aimed at containing these behaviors had better be included in the consultation report. And, obviously, these precipitants are of diagnostic significance as well.

Urgency

In some situations, urgency will be the first issue addressed. This issue should always be made explicit, because there is the danger that the consultee will *assume* that the consultant is aware that the situation is perceived as an emergency and will so respond. The consultee often does not know how to assess the urgency of a psychiatric problem. An offhand comment expressing sadness on the part of a patient may be interpreted as an indication of immediate suicide risk. But incipient delirium tremens, actual suicidal intent, acute organic brain syndromes signaling undiagnosed, treatable complications during the hospital course, and acute paranoia may not be recognized as acutely dangerous conditions that are potentially fatal or disabling to the patient or others. Ask the appropriate diagnostic questions concerning past history of dangerous behavior, sudden onset or exacerbation of confusion or altered state of consciousness, suicidal or homicidal statements or behavior, recent drug or alcohol withdrawal, tremulousness, etc.

If the referring physician does not have this vital information, either he or she or the psychiatrist will have to get it. In the event of a dire consequence, it is little comfort to have stood on ceremony about mechanisms for referrals, schedules, or information required. If there is an emergency, or even a significant likelihood of one, someone will have to see the patient immediately. Emergency measures, such as constant surveillance, may be indicated for the interval until a psychiatrist can appear at the bedside.

It is important to insist in these cases that constant surveillance means that the attendant cannot leave the patient unattended for any reason or for any length of time no matter how short. For example, we have arrived at the room of a patient with an assigned 24-hour "sitter" to find the patient unattended. We discover that the attendant "just made a phone call," "had to go to the bathroom," or "was having a cigarette and a bite to eat." Nonpsychiatric personnel are not aware of the dangerousness, impulsivity, and resourcefulness of some acutely suicidal or psychotic patients.

In many settings, there is a 24-hour call schedule for emergency consultations. In some hospitals with house staff, the resident on call is responsible for seeing patients whose problems are too urgent to wait for a scheduled appointment with the resident and/or attending consultant who have general responsibility for the unit. After receiving a call during working hours, and ascertaining either that the consultee regards the case as an emergency or that there is a significant likelihood of an unrecognized emergency, the regular psychiatric consultant may refer the caller to, or contact, the resident or attending physician on call at that time. Consultation requests after hours and on weekends will go directly to the psychiatrist on call. The system must have been made clear, and agreed upon, in advance.

Location and Availability of Patient

As long as you have a representative of the referring service on the phone, double-check the location of the patient's room. We have spent considerable time tracking a patient from the intensive care unit to the coronary care unit, the step-down unit, and back again. Even the hospital computer is not always up-to-date. It is also wise to ask whether the patient is now, or soon will be, leaving the hospital room for tests, surgery, or other therapeutic procedures. Patients spend a good deal of time in this way, especially during the acute period after admission and the rehabilitation period, at the end of a longer stay.

The clerk on the hospital unit is most likely to be informed about the scheduling of these activities. Gathering information beforehand can save many a fruitless trip. (We also find it useful in many cases to call before making follow-up rounds in order to check that a patient is not at that moment off having a procedure that had not been previously scheduled.) It also may be possible, if your schedule is very tight, to ask that the patient's regimen be changed to allow for your visit. Often, however, such a change would prolong the patient's workup and hospital stay or deprive the patient of a day of treatment such as physical therapy.

As we have stressed in previous chapters, if you decide to go directly to the bedside, and arrive on the hospital unit only to discover that the patient is not there, make some use of the visit. Talk to the staff. Read the chart if it is there; usually, however, it will have gone with the patient. Find a sheet of progress note paper and leave a note to be inserted in the chart when the patient returns. Head it with the title "Preliminary Psychiatric _____ Consultation Note" (fill in the blank with your title: resident or attending, for example) and the date and time. State the reason for the consultation that was communicated to you. State that the patient is not available at this time. Include any information you have gathered from the chart, the staff, the family or visitors present, and the call to the referring physician. Conclude with the date and time you intend to return and information as to where and how you can be reached in the interim.

Determining Who Is the Psychiatrist Responsible for a Given Consultation

In some settings, this is the first question one needs to ask. In others, confusion is infrequent. The patient may belong to an HMO or other plan that determines the need for mental health intervention and supplies its own personnel. In a private-practice setting, the referring physician may have meant to ask a particular private psychiatrist to see the patient, while the service automatically called the hospital consultation service. Or the primary physician may not be aware that the patient has been under the outpatient care of a mental health professional who might be asked to follow the patient through the inpatient stay.

In this latter case, do not assume that this mental health professional can and will address all the patient's psychiatric needs during the hospitalization. The mental health–care provider may not be medically trained, may be a psychiatrist who feels insufficiently expert at dealing with psychiatric issues arising in conjunction with medical illness, or may be unwilling or unable to come to the hospital to tend to the patient during the inpatient stay. In these cases, collaboration between the consultant and the outpatient therapist needs to be carefully planned and executed so as to avoid treatment gaps, confusing duplication of services, and/or conflicting recommendations.

MAKING A CONTRACT FOR THE INITIAL CONSULTATION

Informing the Patient

Ask whether the patient has been asked, or even told, about the planned psychiatric consultation. Generally, we and most other specialists in the field strongly recommend that informing the patient be a required prerequisite for consultation and that an agreement to that effect be part of the negotiations for setting up a consultation service. However, under the best of arrangements, this agreement is sometimes honored in the breach. It is not fair to deprive the patient of the opportunity for an indicated psychiatric assessment because the primary-care service is awkward, punitive, or neglectful about obtaining the patient's consent ahead of time.

If the patient has not been told, try to find out why. Is the patient so oppositional that no one wants to convey any information? Is the responsible physician so busy, on or off the unit, that very little is communicated to the patient about anything? Does the service really feel that because the organic tests were negative, the patient must be hysterical or crazy—but no one wants to say so? Is the patient felt to be incapable of understanding and consenting or refusing? Often, the reason for the failure to inform the patient is the primary physician's affective response. This may be the reason for the consultation as well. All these are extremely useful pieces of clinical information.

How was the need for psychiatric intervention explained to the patient? Having this information can make the patient's initially angry or frightened behavior more understandable. How did the patient react? It helps to know ahead of time when you are likely to have to confront a resentful and/or bewildered patient. Unlike psychiatric office or clinic outpatients, consultation patients have not usually sought psychiatric care on their own or thought of their problems as psychological. Unlike psychiatric inpatients, they may not have serious, well-defined, and obvious psychiatric diseases about which there is a social consensus. They will need emphatic education to make the reason for, and goals of, psychiatric consultation understandable and acceptable (Koran et al. 1979).

The consultant can offer the primary practitioner some suggestions about informing the patient in this initial contact. We find three recommendations most helpful and use them at the bedside ourselves:

1. Relate the reason for consultation to objective observations about the patient—for example, "We notice that you are crying a lot," "You have not been eating," "You sometimes get confused at night and have trouble finding your own room," or "You seem to be seeing upsetting things that the rest of us can't see."
2. Explain that illness is itself stressful. In fact, symptoms for which no explanation can be found can be more stressful than a straightforward diagnosis of disease. Rather than saying, "Since examinations of your gastrointestinal tract are completely negative, the reason for your pain must be in your head," the referring doctor can say, "It is extremely difficult to have a pain, to undergo tests, and to be told that no reason can be found. A psychiatrist, trained in the understanding of both medical and psychological symptoms, can help you cope with this difficult situation."
3. Stress that the psychiatrist is a regular and ongoing part of the medical team, who sees many of the patients on the unit and has had a wide experience in helping medically ill patients. Sometimes staff members, in an effort to decrease their own

and the patient's anxiety, tell the patient that the psychiatric consultant sees every patient on the unit, though this is not the case. Warn the consultee that inaccurate representations of any kind are usually detected by the patient, and undermine trust of the care team and the purpose of the consultation.

Time, Duration, and Content of Initial Consultation

Inform the referring physician when and for how long you plan to perform the initial consultation. Allow yourself latitude to adjust to the clinical realities you encounter at the bedside, within the limits of your own schedule. Make it clear, if such is the case, that successive stages of the consultation will be performed by different members of the consultation team: for example, medical students, residents, nurse practitioners, or other mental health professionals, and attending physicians. If the plans are surprising or unacceptable to your consultee, try to arrive at a compromise or to further clarify the reason for your plan of action.

Discuss what you think you will have to do to make an assessment and arrive at a conclusion in this particular case. If a need is apparent from the initial exchange of information you are having, ask that pertinent medical tests or procedures be performed or ordered while you are arranging to arrive on the floor. Again, leave latitude for unanticipated factors.

Generally, you will plan to review the chart, including history, physical examination, laboratory values, and medication. You may or may not choose to perform your own full or limited physical examination. You will almost certainly talk to staff, and possibly to the patient's family members or friends and acquaintances if they are present. You may ask that the family arrange to be available at the time of your visit. You will conduct an interview with the patient. And you may routinely, or frequently, order related procedures, such as neuropsychological testing. (The performance of these steps is described in subsequent chapters.)

Thus, you now have some idea of what the consultee and the patient want and expect. The referring physician has learned what you want to know, what you would like the patient to know, what you plan to do, and when. Close the conversation by stating when the service can expect to find your consultation note in the

chart and by arranging a time to talk again to discuss your findings and recommendations. Thank the consultee for the referral.

REFERENCES

Balint M: The Doctor, His Patient and the Illness. New York, Interna-
    tional Universities Press, 1957
Borus JF, Casserly NK: Psychiatrists and primary physicians: collabora-
    tive learning experiences in delivering primary care. Hosp Commu-
    nity Psychiatry 30:686–689, 1979
Engel GL: The need for a new medical model. Science 196:129–136, 1977
Glazer WM, Astrachan BM: Social systems approach to consultation-
    liaison psychiatry. Int J Psychiatry Med 9:33–47, 1978–1979
Groves JE: Taking care of the hateful patient. N Engl J Med 298:883–887,
    1978
Kahana RJ, Bibring GL: Personality types in medical management, in
    Psychiatry and Medical Practice in a General Hospital. Edited by Zin-
    berg NE. New York, International Universities Press, 1964,
    pp 108–123
Konior GS, Levine AS: The fear of dying: how patients and their doctors
    behave. Semin Oncol 2:311–316, 1975
Koran LM, Van Natta J, Stephens JR, et al: Patients' reactions to psychi-
    atric consultation. JAMA 241:1603–1605, 1979
Lipowski ZJ: Review of consultation psychiatric and psychosomatic
    medicine. II. Clinical aspects. Psychosom Med 29:201–224, 1967
Meyer E, Mendelson M: Psychiatric consultations with patients on med-
    ical and surgical wards: patterns and processes. Psychiatry
    24:197–220, 1961
Popkin MK, Mackenzie TB: Communicating with the referring physi-
    cian, in Manual of Psychiatric Consultation and Emergency Care.
    Edited by Guggenheim FG, Weiner MF. New York, Jason Aronson,
    1984, pp 115–123
Schiff SK, Pilot ML: An approach to psychiatric care in the general hos-
    pital. Arch Gen Psychiatry 1:349–357, 1959
Strain JJ, Grossman S: Psychological reactions to medical illness and
    hospitalization, in Psychological Care of the Medically Ill. Edited by
    Strain JJ, Grossman S. New York, Appleton-Century-Crofts, 1975,
    pp 23–36
Strain JJ: Psychological Interventions in Medical Practice. New York,
    Appleton-Century-Crofts, 1978

5

The First Visit to the Hospital Unit

The consultant generally goes to the hospital floor at the time agreed upon in the preliminary contact with the referring service. On occasion, it is impossible to discuss the consultation with the primary physician beforehand; when the primary physician cannot be reached, the consultant may decide to proceed with the consultation when convenient, rather than waiting and making a trip to the hospital at a later time. Under these circumstances, in fact, the reasons for contacting the referring physician become reasons for proceeding directly to the hospital unit.

The consultation has been requested because the staff caring for the patient have a psychiatric question that they do not feel competent to answer. They also have limited expertise at judging the urgency of the need for psychiatric intervention. The patient may be suicidal, homicidal, or delirious. The request for consultation is often conveyed by ancillary personnel or house staff who are covering administrative duties but are not knowledgeable about the patient's condition.

The request may be received by members of the psychiatric secretarial staff who are not expert at eliciting, or conveying to the consultant, indications that the need for psychiatric consultation is pressing. In one study, major mental illness was diagnosed twice as often in consultation cases in which the reason for consultation was unclear as in cases in which the reason was clear

(Golinger et al. 1985). When the consultant cannot get reassuring data directly from the physician responsible for the patient and the request, it is best to make this determination for oneself, and as soon as possible after the request is received.

Because of the wide variety of circumstances and procedures for consultation, some consultants may routinely begin consultations on the hospital unit and seek there the information discussed in the previous chapter: the nature of the clinical problem, the patient's general and specific medical condition, the identified psychiatric problem, baseline or premorbid mental status, the degree of familiarity staff have with the patient, the precipitant for calling the consultation, perceived urgency, and whether the consultant or some other psychiatrist should be responsible for the consultation.

The consultant will want to know that the patient has been asked or informed about the consultation, and agreed to be seen. Lastly, before proceeding to see the patient, the consultant will try to establish a preliminary contract with the consultee service as to the timing, methods, and aims of the consultation. If no responsible representative from the service is available for contact, either by telephone or in person, the consultant will indicate his or her view of the contract in the written consultation and/or a conversation with the referring physician after seeing the patient. Whether or not the consultant has made contact with the primary responsible physician, the following issues are addressed and tasks accomplished on the first visit to the hospital unit.

Finding Out Who Is Taking Care of the Patient

In the complex environment of the modern hospital, roles that were traditionally filled by one primary physician are often divided among many members of the staff. This division of labor, sometimes characterized as a fragmentation of care, is relevant to the consultation in at least three ways. First, the continuity and integration of the patient's care may be affected. For example, there may be various staff members writing orders for pharmacologic agents with psychiatric effects and side effects, and still others responsible for making observations of the patient's behavior and symptoms. Chronological correlations between drug administration and clinical change may go unnoticed. Second, the patient may feel confused and insecure about who is responsible for what, and to whom questions and concerns should be addressed. Third, the consultant will need to know to whom observations and suggestions will be most usefully directed (Reichard 1964). The suggestion that one care provider be designated as primary may be one of these suggestions.

Often the most helpful member of the staff in this regard is the head nurse or the patient's "primary nurse," if there is one. Most anyone at the nursing station, especially a clerk or nurse, can identify this person for you (it is often not apparent in the chart). Once you have identified yourself as the psychiatrist who has been asked to consult on the particular patient, ask for the nurse's summary of the case. The following issues should be addressed:

- Who is carrying out various aspects of the patient's care? What have the nurses observed? How does the patient relate to the nursing staff? Are there significant differences in how the patient relates to different nurses? Has the patient confided in, or been most comfortable with, a particular staff member? Has one nurse been identified as most able to deal with the patient?
- How does the patient compare with others who have been hospitalized on the unit with similar conditions? Is the patient more or less ill? Is the patient more or less anxious, depressed, confused, uncooperative? Nurses on a specialty unit acquire considerable depth and breadth of experience in working with patients undergoing the illness or treatment in which the unit specializes (O'Connor and Bilodeau 1987).
- What other personnel have been caring for the patient? Is there, for example, a physical therapist who has been particularly successful in rousing the patient from a state of indifference to work hard at rehabilitation exercises? Does the patient seem particularly upset after trips to the whirlpool for burn debridement? Does the patient seek out the nurse educator who has been assigned to teach newly diagnosed diabetic patients how to manage their blood and urine tests, injections, and diet? Sometimes we have learned that a nursing aide on the midnight shift is the only staff person in whom the patient confides and the most effective at calming and orienting the patient.

The involved nurse can also indicate the roles of the various doctors working with the patient. Who among the involved physicians and physicians-in-training is in closest touch with the patient's progress? Who is following the laboratory values from day to day, making more frequent rounds and physical examinations? Who asks the patient how he or she feels, responds to complaints, and conveys information, plans, and recommendations? This physician will be able to tell you the most about the patient's current status and progress.

Not uncommonly, routine information is imparted by a medical student or house officer, while the attending physician, perhaps less familiar with the ongoing care, only comes to talk to the patient about major or complicated interventions and serious news. This, too, is important information for the consultant. The most senior physician is often (more or less correctly) perceived by the patient as the most expert and powerful member of the medical team. The patient may be upset at the infrequency of contact. Or you may need to enlist this physician's active collaboration if you later make a recommendation, such as psychiatric hospitalization or ECT, that seems weighty or frightening to the patient and family.

In some cases, you may be directly told, or be able to infer, that no one is interacting with the patient very much. It may become clear that no one is interested. A not uncommon situation involves the patient who is elderly, seemingly chronically demented, and without involved relatives to press for active investigation and management. The patient may have been transferred or "dumped" from another service, or admitted by an attending physician who was tired of being harassed by phone calls from the patient and family.

These kinds of clinical situations provoke annoyance and relative psychological neglect on the part of the treating service. There may be so many complications and consultants that no one physician feels capable, or is invested in, overseeing that case as a whole. An illness beyond hope of cure tends to provoke helplessness and withdrawal in the medical staff (Weisman 1975). The fact that the staff members are disinterested for any reason has a powerful influence on the patient's mood, self-esteem, sense of well-being, and expectations, and may well be a factor in whatever signs and symptoms occasioned the request for psychiatric consultation. Increasing staff interest and investment may turn out to be a central part of the process and goal of the consultation.

Attempt to find out which doctor knows the patient best in general. In some hospitals, attending physicians rotate inpatient duties monthly or on some other schedule (Strain 1975). Therefore, there is a good chance that the doctor who had been following the patient before admission is not the doctor responsible for care during the admission. The "real" primary physician may be a member of another specialty who assumed and continued care of the patient on the occasion of an illness episode years ago, a member of the house staff who has been following the patient since an emergency room visit, or an outside physician who referred the patient to the hospital for tertiary care (or the same doctor who is caring for the patient on the current service).

Whoever it is, the doctor who knows the patient best is most likely to be able to tell you the patient's baseline mental status, the patient's usual response to illness, and the past psychiatric history. You may also be able to find out which relatives or friends are likely to be helpful by providing history, spending time with the patient in the hospital, helping the patient think through treatment options, and caring for the patient after discharge.

It may be a different medical staff member who writes the orders in the patient's chart. While in some settings orders may be written by anyone on the staff who is involved in the care of the patient, in others this function is reserved for a physician in one particular role on the service (e.g., the intern). The purpose of this rule is to filter all orders through a final common pathway to avoid redundancy, omissions, and conflicts. At the same time, however, the person who writes the orders may not be the most knowledgeable or involved.

Not uncommonly, the physician responsible for orders is a relatively senior member of the staff who countersigns the orders of a junior house officer or medical student. The countersigning may take place after the order is not only written but carried out, as a routine process removed from the decision making. Because the psychiatric recommendations may well include orders to be carried out, the consultant will need to know the relevant procedure and staff member.

The role of the medical student on a teaching service may well be overlooked by a busy consultant not aware of the practice on a particular unit. Because the active participation of students in the management of patients is a professionally and legally controversial issue, the fact that a student is actually the patient's functional doctor may not be immediately apparent or communicated frankly by the floor staff. The patient is often unaware of the specific roles of the many white-coated practitioners involved in care. The consultant can ask directly about the students' roles on the service, or he or she will learn about these roles after the clerk or nurse helps decipher the signatures on notes and orders in the patient's chart.

STAFF RELATIONSHIPS

The issues of clinical responsibility and order-writing are related to the question of the relationships among medical students, house staff, and attending physicians, as well as other major care providers, on the unit caring for the patient. Dissension or miscommunication among these individuals may well be a factor in the request for consultation. Although it is not stated directly, and may not even be a conscious problem, the consultant is expected to, or needs to, mediate disputes or clarify complex, confusing, and even contradictory approaches and recommendations (Strain 1975).

A patient's suspiciousness and unwillingness to consent to seemingly straightforward interventions may well stem from an awareness that doctors involved in care have differing opinions about what is wrong and how to proceed. The differences may be those of medical style or personality, or may date from a heated conflict in the past or a political rivalry in the present. An example is an oncology unit on which the attending physicians press for aggressive management or research protocols, while some of the house staff are angry and depressed, complaining that patients with no real hope of recovery are pushed into physically painful and otherwise debilitating treatment regimens. Not incidentally, these house staff members are the physicians expected to carry out the treatment plans. Their working schedules also bring them into more close and frequent contact with the patients than do those of the attending physicians. The variance in suggested management may be trivial. However, the emotional undercurrents are easily picked up by the patient, who inwardly concludes that none of the advice is trustworthy, and loses the faith that makes the risks and pain of diagnostic and therapeutic procedures bearable (Lesko et al. 1987).

It is impossible to exaggerate the possibilities for confusion for patients and families confronted with the complexities of a tertiary-care hospital unit. One of the authors hospitalized her own child in the hospital where she worked. With a diagnosis of an unresolving pneumothorax, the child was under the care of the admitting pediatrician, the pediatric surgeon, the specialist in respiratory medicine, and members of the house staff of all three departments. First, it took the family several hours to figure out who was empowered to write an order for a simple analgesic. The next problem was to decide what to do when the surgeon strongly recommended a thoracotomy and the internist insisted it was unnecessary.

Agonizing over the prospect of submitting a child to such major surgery, the author received assurances from each of the specialists that the literature supported his stance. The pediatrician and his partner urged the family to refuse consent for surgery. Finally, the author demanded that the two consultants review the case and the evidence together. One sent a medical student back to the library. It finally appeared that the reason for the reported decrease in recurrence of pneumothorax with repeated episodes was that an increasing number of patients had surgery. This synthesis of information enabled all concerned to agree that an operation was indicated. It was performed and the child is well, 8 years later.

How could a nonmedical family cope with such a situation? It is not uncommon, especially in the kind of setting in which a psychiatric consultant is likely to function and the situations in which the consultant is likely to be called. The resulting confusion, anxiety, depression, rage, passivity/indecision, and/or lack of compliance may indeed precipitate the call for consultation (Strain 1978). The consultant may ameliorate the clinical problem by helping the patient and family clarify the roles and responsibilities of the various care providers (Milano 1982). The physician of record may not be the active primary physician, either because the house staff runs the unit or because a medical complication so dominates the clinical picture that a medical consultant is making the major decisions or recommendations. Lastly, the consultant may want to ask how the patient is getting along with the various members of the team. This is particularly important in cases in which the concern of the consultee is a management problem (e.g., obstreperous behavior with staff or fellow patients, pulling out intravenous lines or feeding tubes, unwillingness to consent). Sometimes it is the very person whose role it is to convey information and orders whom the patient cannot stand.

As mentioned with respect to nurses, it may be possible to identify an ancillary hospital employee whom the patient has befriended and confided in. On several occasions in our experience, a member of the maintenance or catering staff has been able to provide useful information, to suggest how to handle the patient, and/or to actually participate in the management (Freidson 1979). This is particularly true when the employee and patient are members of an ethnic group different from that of the majority of the medical team. These opportunities can be overlooked because staff relations do not facilitate recognition of the roles of nonprofessional staff.

The Patient's Chart

When to Review the Chart

Just as some psychiatrists want full referring information before interviewing a patient, and others feel strongly about forming their own first impressions without preconceptions, some consultants always peruse the chart before the clinical interview and others wait until afterward. The essentials must be obtained at some point before the psychiatric diagnosis and recommendations are made. Not reviewing the chart at all is unacceptable practice, placing the consultant in legal jeopardy (Groves and Vaccarino 1987). We feel that looking at the chart beforehand saves time, because it alerts us to information requiring elucidation in the interview with the patient. However, should the chart not be immediately available when we come to the floor, we do see the patient first.

Overview

The examination of the chart might well be worthy of a chapter or more in itself. However, many of the specifics have to do with laboratory and physical findings characteristic of particular syndromes, conditions, and diseases. These issues are well covered in a variety of other texts focused on psychiatric medicine, consultation, and psychosomatic illness (Hackett and Cassem 1987; Pasnau 1975). For the purposes of this systematic consideration of the consultation process, we will confine ourselves to general issues applicable to any consultation.

The "Old Chart."   The chart is subdivided into components. The charts of patients who have undergone repeated and/or prolonged hospitalizations are often too cumbersome for daily storage and use, so a considerable portion is stored separately or microfilmed. The consultant will have to decide how much time it is feasible to spend going through the old chart in detail. The material is often voluminous and poorly organized, but may contain information of considerable clinical and/or legal significance. Particularly salient points are psychiatric and mental status data.

A patient referred for consultation has sometimes undergone psychiatric evaluation during past hospitalizations as well. The written records are usually the best, or only, structured descriptions of the patient's mental status and psychobehavioral symptoms to be found in the record. These consultations are often entered on color-coded forms, making them easier to locate.

The "Face Sheet."   Most charts have a "face sheet" giving basic demographic information. Of particular interest to the consultant are the next of kin or responsible other, reason for admission, date of admission, employer, and method of payment. The telephone number of the next of kin or person who accompanied the patient to the hospital enables the consultant to call this person, who usually knows the patient well, is committed to his or her well-being, and may be central to discharge planning.

The kind of work the patient does, and the fact that the patient was or was not employed before admission, are clues to level of function, possible work stress, and exposure to toxins and other factors in the workplace that have a bearing on the patient's medical and psychiatric condition. The patient's insurance coverage, public assistance status if any, and financial status will probably have a major impact not only on the patient's biopsychosocial condition but also on the options available for psychiatric care and follow-up. Many consultants would prefer to be aware of these options, or lack of them, when they begin working with the staff and patient.

Admission Notes.   The admission notes generally contain the most complete histories and results of physical examinations, as well as summaries of past medical events and recent medical interactions. While the consultant cannot rely on the admitting physician to have summarized all relevant data from the old chart and current informants, the choice and content of information is important. Be alert for indications of baseline and admitting mental status, and changes in this status. Note relevant physical findings so that you can determine whether they were followed up. For example, there may be clues that the patient is thyrotoxic, suffering from an infectious process, or pregnant. Has there been untreated substance abuse? Withdrawal states are common in the general hospital population. Note whether there are ongoing or new signs that the prognosis is worsening, dire, or "hopeless," or that staff is at a loss how to manage a refractory illness, deal with the patient's personality style, or help the patient control an addiction or other self-defeating behavior.

The admission notes are another source for the names of the patient's friends or relatives whom you may wish to contact. There may also be indications of past and current levels of psychosocial functioning. Are the findings for which consultation is requested spelled out? And does the overall tone and content of the written workup indicate the level of the writer's interest in, and knowledge of, the patient as an individual and as a part of the family and other social systems?

Progress Notes.   Note when signs and symptoms of the identified psychiatric problem are first entered in the record. Were they correlated with changes in physical or laboratory findings, views of prognosis, or treatments administered? How is the patient doing in general? When is discharge anticipated? Is impending or delayed discharge a precipitant for psychiatric consultation? What specific discharge plans and problems exist? The patient's psychiatric symptoms may be a manifestation of fears of life outside the hospital or fears he or she will never get out. Plans of nursing home placement or other moves, the thought of imposing on overburdened relatives, or the prospect of managing alone may be upsetting the patient. And how long does the consultant have to make an assessment, develop a relationship with the patient, begin psychiatric care under hospital observation, and make follow-up arrangements, before the patient leaves the unit? Which doctor(s) is following the patient daily?

Nursing and Other Staff Notes. The nursing notes are parallel to those of the medical staff, but from a different perspective. They may include mention of specifics of the mental status, such as quotations of the patient's complaints, requests, and unusual verbal productions (e.g., descriptions of delusions and hallucinations). They track important psychobiological parameters such as sleep and food intake. The nurses may note what visitors the patient had, unusual behavior of visitors, and reactions of the patient to visits. This information about visitors is often very helpful. It leads the consultant to useful historians and collaborators and provides a clue to interactions that may be precipitating problematic episodes.

For example, the patient may be soothed and cooperative while a relative is present, desolate when a relative leaves, angry and agitated with another visitor, or sad or homesick because visits are rare. There may be indications that visitors are supplying the patient with illicit substances such as alcohol or street drugs, or threatening the patient with violence. There may be "unfinished business" stemming from an attack or confrontation that led to the assault or self-injury responsible for the hospitalization.

Vital Signs. Note the absolute values and course of the patient's vital signs. Blood pressure, pulse rate and rhythm, respiratory rate and rhythm, and temperature are, indeed, "vital" indications of the patient's general condition and specific response to the disease process and medical interventions. Clarify whether there is any correlation between episodes of confusion or disorientation and transient deviations in these values.

Perhaps there are runs of tachycardia or spells of respiratory depression causing cerebral hypoxia.

Laboratory Values and Other Test Results.   Unfortunately, the consultant cannot assume that the results of blood chemistry, blood gas, radiologic, ultrasound, computed tomography, magnetic resonance, electroencephalographic, electromyographic, and electrocardiographic tests, and all the others, will be neatly extracted and summarized in the progress notes and used effectively in the diagnostic and therapeutic process. One of the functions of a consultant is to offer a separate and fresh overview and approach to a medical problem. The consultant may discover an overlooked laboratory value that confirms a diagnosis or condition explaining or contributing to the patient's behavioral aberrations. It has been estimated that 20% to 50% of patients with physical illnesses suffer from psychiatric illnesses, and vice versa (Lipowski 1975).

Often, a patient suffers from a combination of moderate, but significant, deficits that in sum can account for a delirium (Slaby and Cullen 1987). For example, the patient is anemic, hypoxic, febrile, and has an elevated ammonia level. A surgical record may reveal dips in blood pressure, or episodes of cardiovascular collapse that compromise the postoperative mental status in a patient whose baseline cerebral function was borderline. Needless to say, postulating a link between a medical/surgical procedure or oversight and an adverse outcome raises issues of diplomacy at the least and of medical malpractice at the worst.

Other Consultations.   Have a look at the findings and opinions of other specialists who have been asked to see the patient. You will learn how various other consultants view not only the patient but also the consultation process. There will be differing or confirmatory assessments of the physical findings and laboratory values, and often different pieces and views of the history, depending on when it was obtained, by whom, and from whom. The spectrum of specialties involved will be another indication of how the primary service conceptualizes the clinical problem. A large number of consultations suggests both a complex problem and a primary service unwilling and/or unable to deal with it. The many consultations have also probably been exhausting and confusing to the patient and have conveyed the message that the doctors in charge are impressed, not to say overwhelmed, by the difficulty of the case.

Consultations also may indicate the general level of care of the patient before hospitalization, the concern of the service for the patient's general well-being, and/or the patient's level of demands or feelings of entitlement. Some patients who have been neglected before admission will have been seen by the hospital dentist, ophthalmologist, dermatologist, etc., for chronic conditions, because this care has not been available to them on an outpatient basis. This information will help the psychiatric consultant evaluate the degree to which a patient's affective or psychotic disorder or psychosocial circumstances have interfered with his or her self-care.

VISITORS

Often, visitors—friends, relatives, members of the clergy—are at the bedside or on the floor when the consultant arrives. Rather than simply asking them to wait outside when it is time to interview the patient, the consultant should ask them to spare a moment to offer information. The consultant cannot offer information to them without the permission of the patient. In fact, the fact that a psychiatrist has been called in could be construed as privileged, and is, in at least one state (Illinois, General Assembly 1988). But there is no limitation on what the visitors can tell the staff, including the consultant. The presence of visitors at the interview and negotiations with the patient about the consultant's interactions with them will be discussed in the next chapter.

In this first encounter, the consultant might ask the visitors how they are related to the patient and how well they know him or her. The specific nature of their relationship is relevant. For example, an adult child of a confused elderly patient may assert that the parent was mentally clear and independent before the hospitalization. The consultant inquires closely about the nature of their interactions and learns that the relative has not spent a significant amount of time with the patient in months. In another case, the minister may just shake hands with the patient after each Sunday service and make a polite pastoral call in the hospital, or may work closely with the patient on a church committee, observing the patient doing exemplary work on an intellectually demanding task.

Next find out how the patient's current affective and cognitive state and personality style compare with those familiar to the visitor. A state that seems perfectly understandable to staff who do not know the patient may nevertheless be so much at variance with the patient's baseline as to warrant diagnostic and/or therapeutic intervention. For example, we were consulted about an elderly man who had a stroke. He was hardly speaking or relating to staff. He ate little and sloppily. His grooming was poor. The neurology service wondered whether he was depressed, whether his signs and symptoms derived purely from his organic deficit, or whether he had a preexisting impairment. No relatives could be reached. The patient's address was in a minority neighborhood bordering on a slum. The patient said almost nothing in response to our questions and dribbled his food on his hospital gown when he was encouraged to eat a few bites. We were leaving his room, not much enlightened, when we encountered an elegantly dressed man on his way in. We asked to speak to him. He turned out to be a physician and close friend of the patient. He informed us that the patient was a cultured and previously immaculate retired school principal and opera buff, who, his friend was sure, would react to any compromise of his dignity with a profound depression.

Before leaving the visitors, find out where they can be reached if you need to contact them at a future time. Let them know where to reach you if they think of other information you should have. Allow them, time permitting, to voice their concerns, questions, observations, theories, and suggestions. Let them know that you cannot answer their questions until the patient has given permission and the case has been discussed with the primary physician, but that you will be happy to talk to them when these negotiations have been completed. They might be willing to wait until you have finished the initial consultation. You may well have additional questions after you have interviewed the patient.

Conclusions

A substantial amount of work on the consultation can be accomplished before the patient is even seen. Especially with medically ill patients—who may be too physically exhausted, confused, or neurologically depressed, respiratorily compromised, or busy with procedures off the unit, to give a full medical and psychiatric history—information from hospital personnel, visitors, and the hospital chart is extremely valuable. Forearmed with all available information about the patient's past and current state, and the questions and concerns of others involved in the patient's life and care, the consultant can target the available interview time more specifically to answering the consultee's question(s) and making a well-reasoned diagnostic and management formulation.

References

Freidson E: Conflicting perspectives in the hospital, in Health, Illness, and Medicine: A Reader in Medical Sociology. Edited by Albrecht GL, Higgins PC. Chicago, IL, Rand McNally, 1979, pp 292–296

Golinger R, Teitelbaum ML, Folstein MF: Clarity of request for consultation: its relationship to psychiatric diagnosis. Psychosomatics 26:649–653, 1985

Groves JE, Vaccarino JM: Legal aspects of consultation, in Massachusetts General Hospital Handbook of General Hospital Psychiatry, 2nd Edition. Edited by Hackett TP, Cassem NH. Littleton, MA, PSG Publishers, 1987, pp 591–617

Hackett TP, Cassem NH (eds): Massachusetts General Hospital Handbook of General Hospital Psychiatry, 2nd Edition. Littleton MA, PSG Publishers, 1987

Illinois, General Assembly: Mental Health and Developmental Disabilities Confidentiality Act, PA80-1508, 1988

Lesko LM, Massie MJ, Holland JC: Oncology, in Principles of Medical Psychiatry. Edited by Stoudemire MD, Fogel BS. Orlando, FL, Grune & Stratton, 1987, pp 495–520

Lipowski ZJ: Psychiatry of somatic diseases: epidemiology, pathogenesis, classification. Compr Psychiatry 16:105–124, 1975

Milano MR: The management of family and marital problems, in Psychiatric Management for Medical Practitioners. Edited by Kornfeld DS, Finkel JB. New York, Grune & Stratton, 1982, pp 168–184

O'Connor S, Bilodeau CB: The psychiatric nurse clinical specialist in liaison psychiatry, in Massachusetts General Hospital Handbook of

General Hospital Psychiatry. Edited by Hackett TP, Cassem NH. Littleton, MA, PSG Publishers, 1987, pp 572–590

Pasnau RO (ed): Consultation-Liaison Psychiatry. New York, Grune & Stratton, 1975

Reichard JF: Teaching principles of medical psychology to medical house officers, in Psychiatry and Medical Practice in a General Hospital. Edited by Zinberg NE. New York, International Universities Press, 1964, pp 169–204

Slaby AE, Cullen LO: Dementia and delirium, in Principles of Medical Psychiatry. Edited by Stoudemire MD, Fogel BS. Orlando, FL, Grune & Stratton, 1987, pp 135–175

Strain JJ: The anatomy of the teaching hospital, in Psychological Care of the Medically Ill. Edited by Strain JJ, Grossman S. New York, Appleton-Century-Crofts, 1975, pp 171–184

Strain JJ: Psychological Interventions in Medical Practice. New York, Appleton-Century-Crofts, 1978

Weisman AD: The dying patient, in Consultation-Liaison Psychiatry. Edited by Pasnau RO. New York, Grune & Stratton, 1975, pp 237–244

6

Seeing the Patient

After discussing the case and preliminary contract with the referring physician, talking with hospital staff and visitors who know the patient, and reviewing the chart, the consultant goes to the bedside to interview the patient. The preparation to be described may be much more intense and complex than the preliminaries that the consultant undertakes with other sorts of patient interactions (Lipowski 1967). With an outpatient who has chosen to seek psychiatric care, the negotiations are generally limited to the psychiatrist-patient dyad. A consultation involves at least the triad of primary physician–consultant–patient and often is more complicated, involving others who identified the need for consultation, who know the patient, who are having problems with management, and/or who are involved with the patient's care, either professionally or personally.

This unique situation has an impact on the patient's attitude toward the consultation (Meyer and Mendelson 1961). The general-hospital inpatient for whom consultation has been requested has not usually initiated the decision that a psychiatrist is required for his or her care. Sometimes there is an active request or enthusiastic acceptance of the suggestion; more often there is passive acceptance, grudging compliance, or more or less assertive reluctance (Koran et al. 1979). The patient has not prepared for the consultation. And the medically ill patient's ability to cooperate is limited by debilitating physical symptoms of the particular illness; preoccupation and fear about the medical condition, treatment, and prognosis; and general malaise and weakness (Dvoredsky and Cooley 1986).

The consultation situation can also facilitate the patient's psychological availability to the psychiatrist. The same exhaustion that limits the ability to engage in a new relationship also tends to lower psychological defenses. Being alone, frightened, and in unfamiliar surroundings enhances the likelihood that the patient will relate to and appreciate a professional who is interested and expert in dealing with feelings as well as knowledgeable about physical illness (Strain 1975). Crises are times when people can stagnate, regress, or grow; old patterns are susceptible to rearrangement. The interview conducted under these circumstances has to be focused; it may have to be brief or conducted in several brief parts because of the patient's exhaustion or other clinical interruptions. Nevertheless, the need for decisions about psychiatric interventions may be immediate. These and a number of other factors to be clarified and addressed below are particularly characteristic of the consultation interview.

UNIQUE ISSUES IN PSYCHIATRIC CONSULTATION

Patient Consent and Preparation

There are patients who ask, and even demand, to see a mental health professional or a psychiatrist in particular. Some of these patients have had previous positive experiences with psychopharmacologic and/or psychotherapeutic interventions. Others feel themselves to be under overwhelming stress or to be experiencing symptoms they identify as psychiatric, such as anxiety, affective illness, or psychosis. Other patients accept the idea as a sensible suggestion. Many others are mystified, put off, frightened, or insulted. A great deal depends upon the explicit and implicit messages conveyed to the patient by the primary care provider.

One common instance involves the patient upon whom a huge array of laboratory tests and examinations have been performed in an unavailing effort to make sense of a symptom complex and to identify a "medically" treatable medical condition. The primary physician, confirmed in the impression that the patient is a "crock" or somatizer, conveys the negative workup results to the patient with great conviction and perhaps some disdain. On the eve of hospital discharge, the physician goes on to explain that because the problem is now obviously "in your head," there is "nothing more the service can offer," and that the psychiatrist will be by presently. This introduction handicaps the consultant. But this classic situation can have positive effects on the psychiatric consultation. The patient may be more likely to respond to a new physician when the therapeutic alliance with the referring physician is in jeopardy.

Even when not actively averse to the psychiatric consultation, the patient will not have undergone the same introspective affective and cognitive process as does the patient who works through a decision to seek psychiatric help. The general-hospital patient is less likely to have noticed repeated patterns of problematic behavior and poor life outcomes, symptoms that recur under specific life conditions, or a family history of similar complaints. Consultation patients often have not realized that tearfulness, sleeplessness, feelings of helplessness, or changes in interpersonal behavior styles are psychiatric symptoms. (Techniques for handling this consultation situation are discussed below.) It is rare that the expert consultant cannot persuade a patient to engage in an initial interview.

Confidentiality

Traditionally, communications between psychiatrist—or any doctor—and patient have been privileged and confidential in medical ethics and under United States law. In recent years, court decisions and legislation have impinged on this absolute rule. Rules vary among states, and contradictory regulations and court decisions may coexist in the same state. For example, state agencies may be empowered to examine patients' charts to determine the need for or quality of care. At the same time, in Illinois, for example, the current Mental Health and Developmental Disabilities Confidentiality Act specifies that even the fact that a patient has been psychiatrically hospitalized may not be a part of that patient's medical record (Illinois, General Assembly 1988). Psychiatrists and nonpsychiatrists alike are frustrated by the need to

care for patients when vital information such as current psychopharmacologic treatment is not in the medical chart.

Younger psychiatrists may not be aware that the privilege of
confidentiality traditionally belongs to the patient and not to the
doctor. That is, the patient may choose to release the records of
the diagnostic or therapeutic contact. Some psychiatrists who do
understand this interpretation of confidentiality do not consider it
sound psychiatric practice; they feel that the knowledge that the
communications may not be kept completely confidential interferes with a patient's ability to participate fully in the therapeutic
process and prejudices other persons in the community who are
considering psychiatric referral.

Psychiatric consultation does not allow for this traditional
model of confidentiality. Although many physicians may have
taken the exchange of medical information among professional
members of a hospital staff for granted, consent for the forward-
ing of records from one medical office or institution to another
requires written consent of the patient. Information vital to the
patient's safety or survival may be exchanged (American Psychiatric Association 1985). There is good reason for careful control of
the dissemination of psychiatric data: cases in which information
about a patient is bandied about as gossip or used to label the
patient pejoratively. But an inhibition on the free exchange of
information about a patient can also be problematic.

For example, one of the authors (N.L.S.) was asked to see a
patient after an exploratory operation performed in an effort to
improve the patient's fertility revealed that her fallopian tubes
were beyond repair. The patient, who held a doctorate and a professional position in another field, had initially informed the surgeon that she wished to have his opinion because she was dissatisfied with the care provided by her previous doctor. She insisted
that there be no contact between them. She asserted that she was
fully informed about her condition and could give the new doctor,
from whom she expected better results, all necessary information. In the course of the physical examination, she explained that
a scar on her breast was the result of an excisional biopsy of a
benign mass. She underwent the exploration, and upon waking
from the anesthesia and being informed of the findings, she
demanded that the doctor not tell anyone else, including her
husband.

The former doctor was passing the nursing station one day soon after this operation, and recognizing the patient's name on a chart, she rushed to tell the current physician that she had been extremely concerned about this patient. The mass removed from the breast a few months before had been malignant. The patient had refused any form of care of the cancer and had forbidden the doctor to inform her family of the diagnosis; she was certain that her husband's parents would convince him to divorce her if they believed she could not bear him children. Had the second operation been successful, the patient might have conceived a pregnancy while suffering from a malignancy. Possibly surgery of any kind had been an additional risk under the circumstances. The patient threatened to sue the surgeon if she told anyone about the malignancy or the infertility.

The present doctor made a bargain with this patient. He agreed to respect her wishes for confidentiality if she would see a psychiatrist. He hoped the consultant would be able to discover and treat the profound and seemingly irrational anxiety that was leading the patient to endanger her life by refusing treatment. The patient was enraged; she cooperated only in the most superficial way, and explicitly under duress, with the consultation. The consultation, under these conditions, was a fruitless exercise. The patient vehemently denied all psychiatric signs, symptoms, and history and defended the reasoning behind her decision. No decrements in cognitive function could be demonstrated. The patient left the hospital, never to contact any of the involved physicians again.

The consultant decided that the confidentiality the patient had insisted on in this case had been detrimental to her care. We would prefer to insist on the free exchange of information among doctors involved in the care of any patient we see. It is conceivable that this principle would have to be compromised in an initial, urgent consultation—on a paranoid patient, for example—but it is a useful principle nonetheless.

Consultations are performed under the assumption that the primary physician will be informed of the findings. It is the primary physician, not the patient, who is the consultee. In a general-hospital setting, many other persons involved in the patient's care will actively seek, be actively informed of, or be exposed to the results of the consultation. Some, like third-party payers and utilization reviewers, may read it without therapeutic intent. Nevertheless, the presumption of privilege cannot be abandoned without notice or negotiation.

In the interest of honesty and a working alliance, the consultant should inform the patient of the primary physician's question, the purpose of the consultation, and the fact that the contents and conclusions of the interview will be entered in the chart and discussed with members of the medical-care team. When indicated, state that there is a medical obligation to reveal and act on information indicating that the patient is in immediate danger of some kind, typically of suicide or homicide. Add that, at the conclusion of the interview, the consultant and patient can discuss any items that the patient would prefer not be revealed. It sometimes happens that certain specifics of the patient's history (e.g., an extramarital affair) are significant for psychiatric diagnosis and therapy but embarrassing to the patient and inessential for the primary physician. The consultant can keep private notes for purposes of completeness, and to have available as a memory aid for future reference, without entering every item into the official written consultation. Some consultation services maintain a file of these documents under lock and key in the psychiatry department, where they can be used for reference in future consultations and/or research. The consultation note in the chart must be focused and relatively brief in any case (see Chapter 8 of this manual; Garrick and Stotland 1982).

The Contract—Conflicts

The confidentiality question is one aspect of the peculiar nature of a consultation, in which the psychiatrist's contract is, initially at least, with a patient's doctor and not with the patient. Clearly, at some time in the consultation process there develops a duty to, and contract with, the patient as well. The triadic nature of this interaction comes into the foreground at the time of the live interaction with the patient. Not only is information shared with the primary-care team, but the observation and interpretation of interactions among the patient and various members of the team not infrequently become part of the consultation.

The patient may complain of unsatisfactory treatment by one or another care provider and attribute emotional or behavioral signs and symptoms to this perceived inadequacy: "Wouldn't you be angry if no nurse came for an hour after you rang for a bedpan?" "I will not consent to surgery recommended by some young intern." "I guess I am depressed because my doctor hardly ever comes by, and when she does she has no time to talk to me." These patient complaints are psychiatric data. Like all patient statements, they can arouse powerful feelings in the psychiatrist and must be subject to interpretation and corroboration as appropriate. The consultant will look for substantiating or controverting evidence, weigh the objective validity of the complaints, and then decide how to help all concerned, in the interest of the patient. In some situations, the psychiatrist will note imperfections in care that the patient has not complained of or that the patient has consciously or unconsciously precipitated. There may be, as noted in the preceding chapter, conflicts among members of the staff, the consequences of which are revealed directly or indirectly in the interview (Glazer and Astrachan 1978–1979).

The interview may also reveal character disorders that make the patient difficult for anyone, including the consultant, to deal with (Kahana and Bibring 1964). One can begin to formulate suggestions to help the service cope (Groves 1975). The consultant must navigate between being perceived by the staff as the patient's agent, and by the patient as the staff's agent, to function and be regarded as an interpreter and facilitator.

Conduct of the Interview

Technical Questions

Some aspects of the technique of the interview are functions of the unique situation of consultation. A specific effort must be made to enlist the patient's understanding and collaboration. The physical and logistical arrangements may be daunting. The consultant must be prepared to find the patient in the process of bathing, using the bedpan, or undergoing a medical procedure, and must use pragmatic tact to decide when to wait, step aside, or assert the need to interrupt so as to perform the interview. If the room is shared with other patients, draw the curtains between the beds for the time being. They are ineffective as a sound barrier, but the gesture demonstrates respect for the patient's privacy and is meaningful. Corroborate the patient's name. Mistaken identity and changes of rooms are common in hospitals. Introduce yourself by name.

Dealing with visitors is a delicate matter. The patient may feel more comfortable during the interview with a close friend or relative in attendance. Also, the visitor may have valuable information to communicate, may help the patient remember items from the history, and may be stimulated by the interview to notice discrepancies, omissions, and deviations from the patient's usual cognitive and affective state. However, the very fact that a psychiatrist has been called in consultation is confidential between patient and staff. Should the patient not wish a visitor to know about it, even an introduction in a visitor's presence may be a breach of confidentiality.

The consultant will have to assess each clinical situation and the available time for subtleties. The optimal course is to ask the visitor to wait nearby, and then introduce oneself to the patient and ask whether he or she prefers to be interviewed with or without the visitor. At the conclusion of the interview, ask the patient whether it is acceptable that you speak to the visitor, alone and/or in the patient's presence.

Not only visitors but also hospital staff members and other patients may intrude upon the privacy of the consultation interview. If the patient is ambulatory, or can be safely conveyed by wheelchair, and there is a private lounge or examining, treatment, or conference room on the unit, you may want to offer the patient the option of interviewing there. When that is not possible, the patient will appreciate your acknowledgement of the importance of privacy. The interview can almost always proceed without significant inhibition by the unavoidable presence of others. It may be necessary to ask that the television or radio be turned down, other conversations be conducted quietly, etc.

Often, as mentioned above, a consultation patient's ability to engage in the interview is compromised by the medical condition. The patient's self-esteem and sense of identity are impaired by the situation: lying in bed, clad in a hospital gown, with modesty limited by the need for catheters, traction, airing of bedsores, etc. The patient may be intubated, too weak to talk for more than a few minutes, interrupted by coughing, or distracted by physical pain. We have even arrived at the bedside to find the patient "in extremis" and have called for the resuscitation team. Such situations put the consultant's responsibility as a physician in bold relief.

The patient's discomfort also gives the psychiatric consultant the opportunity to demonstrate the basic human compassion and helpfulness that are the basis for the therapeutic alliance (Finkel 1982). If the patient needs a tissue, a bedpan, help finding a more comfortable position, or help reaching the bedside tray or ringing telephone, do not proceed with an interview without attending to this need. Handing the patient a tissue or locating the nurse to bring a bedpan or analgesic is in many cases the beginning of a trusting doctor-patient relationship with a skeptical patient (Yager 1989).

Explaining the Consultant's Presence: Relieving Anxiety and Soliciting Cooperation

After introductions, privacy, and comfort are attended to, elicit and deal with the patient's understanding of, and reaction to, your presence. Fostering the cooperation of an unenthusiastic or unwilling patient involves the essence of psychiatric knowledge and skill. Explain that you are a psychiatrist who has been asked by the primary service or doctor to see the patient. Observe the patient's reaction. If the patient says, "Oh, good, I was expecting you. I'm going crazy with anxiety," you can proceed with your usual interview, taking the other factors discussed in this chapter into account. If the patient appears surprised, confused, angry, or otherwise upset by the prospect of psychiatric consultation, that feeling must be attended to. Focusing on and using the patient's affect is the core of a meaningful dialogue.

When the patient is surprised or angry, complaining that there has been no communication from the primary physician about the consultation request, the consultant had best express understanding about how disconcerting that must be. You may leave the bedside and attempt to contact the primary physician to request that he or she explain the reason for the consultation and obtain the patient's consent. However, most consultants prefer to get on with the interview once they have come to the hospital floor and to explore the patient's complaint of failure to obtain consent in the course of the consultation. In some cases, the patient will have forgotten, suppressed, or repressed an interaction on the subject that did take place.

We immediately ground the reason for consultation in consensual reality by explaining what observable behavior of the patient concerned the primary physician: "Your doctor is worried because you haven't been eating—appeared confused last night—are having a hard time making up your mind about the proposed surgery—seem so nervous that you can't get any rest—are having trouble because you hear voices." If there is no indication in the chart or from any of the people involved with the patient that psychosis is a diagnostic consideration, we may add: "Some people think that psychiatrists only come to see crazy people. Your doctor does not think you are crazy." This reassurance addresses a very common fear and enables the patient to engage in the diagnostic process.

Next we explain that we function as part of the regular hospital team, working with the psychological issues and stresses of patients on that particular service. This is additional relief, and the patient may at this point be willing or even eager to discuss the painful psychiatric symptoms. Some patients, however, retort that what is bothering them is their physical symptoms and, perhaps, the failure of the primary treatment team to successfully diagnose and allay them.

The consultant will then probably want to take a history of the physical symptoms. This procedure serves several functions. It demonstrates to the patient the psychiatrist's genuine interest in the problem that most concerns the patient (MacKinnon and Michels 1971). It also underscores the psychiatrist's medical identity and knowledge, and it may well reveal chronologies, repetitions, anniversaries, and other clues to the psychological meanings of physical illness to the patient (Kimball 1969). If the patient is irate at any implication of psychological etiology, explain that it is stressful to have symptoms that no one has been able to understand or eliminate. We take a neutral stance on psychological etiology, underscoring the fact that the mind-brain and body are intrinsically interactive. We offer examples such as "bleeding ulcers," a "real" physical disease commonly acknowledged to be related to stress, or the "butterflies in the stomach" experienced by most people stressed by having to perform. "In any case," we state, "we will try to help in whatever way we can." We add that perhaps the patient will discover that some life situation is playing a role in the illness and that perhaps we can help with the impact of the illness on the life situation.

The Patient Who Refuses Psychiatric Interview

Once in a great while, a patient will flatly refuse to talk to the consultant. It would be simplest to end the consultation there, declaring that the patient has the right to refuse this intervention like any other. But the consultation may have been requested because the patient's verbal or nonverbal behavior suggested a risk of suicide or homicide, an organic brain syndrome possibly symptomatic of a life-threatening complication, or a delusional inability to make rational decisions about medical treatment (Colon et al. 1988). In these cases, the hospital and consultant would be remiss to simply honor the patient's demand that the psychiatrist leave. And, in our experience, it is precisely these very ill patients at risk who are the few who do refuse.

In these cases, we consider very carefully all the information we have gathered so far from the staff, chart, family, etc. If there is a question of necessity for psychiatric inpatient commitment or for obtaining a guardian to make medical decisions, and the patient seems able, but unwilling, to participate in the psychiatric evaluation, we sometimes say, in language the patient can understand: "The information conveyed to me by your doctor means that you may be at risk unless you are committed to a psychiatric unit—have surgery against your will [or whatever the particular concern]. Therefore, if you do not talk to me and give me evidence to controvert what I have been told, I may be forced to assume that you need this protection."

Most patients who are able will respond to this straightforward confrontation. If the patient does not respond and does not have any apparent medical condition inhibiting communication, the consultant will have to draw on other sources of information to determine how to proceed. If there has been no indication of danger, the consultant might just withdraw, explain in a written note what has happened, and decide on the next step in collaboration with the primary-care team. The consultee may want to offer the patient an enhanced explanation for the consultation, or he or she may prefer to drop the matter of interview for the time being. The consultant and consultee may agree to confer about the case using other sources of information.

If there are indications that the verbally uncommunicative patient may have a functional or organic psychosis and/or a risk of harming himself or herself, or others, protective measures such as 24-hour surveillance, commitment, or guardianship may have to be instituted. The consultant's note in the chart will explain the careful reasoning process and expert psychiatric judgment that supported the decision (Mills and Daniels 1987). Explain them in person to the patient as well, whether or not the patient appears to be able to understand or respond.

Interview Content

Of the spectrum of interview styles, the most appropriate for the average consultation situation is the crisis intervention or brief psychotherapy model (Bellak and Small 1965). Psychodynamic understanding is necessary, but the circumstances do not allow the time for a spontaneous exposition of many hours. Even if the patient is well enough and willing to talk, his or her preoccupation is likely to be with the medical condition that is necessitating the ongoing hospitalization.

Psychiatrists vary in their opinions about allowing somatizing patients (one subgroup of the consultant's practice) to dwell on their symptoms in ongoing psychotherapy. But most psychiatrists who function as general-hospital consultants agree that it is essential that hospital patients be allowed and encouraged to express their physical concerns, and that the psychiatrist take a genuine interest in them, at the time of the initial interview. When an illness—or symptoms—is severe enough to require the patient to leave the familiar surroundings of home and work, give up ordinary gratifications and productivity, and relocate to the alien conditions and often painful interventions of the hospital, the illness or symptoms are the patient's major preoccupation (Kimball 1981).

The contents of the standard medical history outline, as applied in the consultation setting (see Chapter 8), include chief complaint, history of present illness, review of systems, past history, social history (including education, employment, antisocial behavior, and relationships), family history, current medications and other treatments, and habits relevant to health. This outline is known to, and practiced by, all physicians (Rogers and Rasof 1977). Its use reinforces medical identity and underscores the intrinsic indivisibility of phenomena artificially, but traditionally, divided into "psychological" and "somatic." A "routine" medical history, including both somatic and psychological (emotional) symptoms, allows for the elaboration of the psychodynamic issues, premorbid condition, and important specific pieces of data.

What has been the patient's characteristic personality style and response to illness and other unusual demands? Under what life circumstances do symptoms appear, become exacerbated, or abate, and what does the patient do to promote these outcomes? What, as precisely as possible, precipitated the current episode? How have the hospitalization and care been experienced (Weisman 1987)?

How have significant others responded? Does the patient feel that things have been getting better or worse? What does the patient feel is wrong, and what measures does the patient think should be taken? Have there been similar episodes in the patient or in significant others, and how have they been treated and resolved? What are the specifics of previous interactions with mental health professionals (diagnosis, drugs and dosages, response, reason for ending contact)? Something related to the hospitalization is generally the precipitant and/or chief complaint.

For purposes of clarity of thinking, reimbursement by third-party payers, standardization, and communication with the primary-care physician and others, including future psychiatric consultants, the psychiatric consultant today usually must make a DSM-III-R and/or ICD-9-CM diagnosis. Although the individual psychiatrist may take issue with the philosophy, style, or content of all or part of DSM-III-R, it is the accepted diagnostic reference of the day and offers a standardized phenomenological approach to psychiatric illness. In any case, the explicit use of a particular diagnostic system informs and structures the interview.

Mental Status Examination

It is not our purpose here to explicate the performance of the mental status examination, but to clarify issues that come up in the context of consultation. There is some expressed and/or latent controversy in our field about the necessity and usefulness of the formal mental status examination. Perhaps in all psychiatric interviews, but certainly in consultations, it is essential to elicit, record, and base diagnostic and therapeutic opinions on an organized, systematic account of the particulars of the patient's cognitive and affective state. This account is a vital reference point in comparisons with past and future findings. It may include the following:

- Appearance
- Level of consciousness
- Orientation
- Cooperation
- Behavior: motor and verbal
- Affect
- Relatedness to interviewer
- Thought content
- Cognition: memory (immediate, short-term, long-term); calculation; intelligence; fund of information; abstraction; insight; judgment; concentration
- Psychotic symptoms
- Suicidality/homicidality

Both the findings at the time of interview and the course of the mental status are central factors in the differential diagnosis and the evaluation of the response to changes in medical condition and/or therapy. The psychiatrist's mental status examination also serves as a model for the other health-care professionals who observe it. It is an example of the performance of the examination, and it demonstrates the status of the particular patient at the time. The discrepancy between the assumptions they have drawn from their briefer and less systematic interaction and the deficits or strengths the patient demonstrates on formal examination can be quite striking.

Both the technique and the importance of the mental status

examination are underemphasized in most health-care education. Most professionals probably cannot usefully recall its components, and feel uncomfortable asking a patient these types of questions. The observation of a consultant imparts knowledge and skills without forcing a revelation of the awkwardness felt by these individuals. This is particularly important in view of the fact that a large proportion of hospital patients suffer from acute and/or chronic organic brain syndromes (Murray 1987).

A skilled interviewer can elicit reproducible, objective mental status information from many patients without doing a formal mental status examination. The date, time, place, and person can be woven into the dialogue. The patient's affective state, flow of thought, judgment and insight, ability to concentrate, etc., can all be evident in an interview. However, if no formal process is pursued, the interviewer must exercise particular care that no element of the examination is overlooked. The formal exam is a methodical, condensed technique for obtaining and recording the same information. Condensed (or "mini") mental status examinations have also been developed in an effort to shorten the process, decrease patient and examiner discomfort, and focus on questions that have been demonstrated to have validity (Kahn 1960).

Like all medical interviewers, the psychiatric consultant will focus on the areas of the examination that appear to be most crucial and revealing as data emerge. How would the medical problems of which the patient complains be likely to affect mental status? Mental status aberrations appearing in the interview can also lead the consultant to suspect a previously undisclosed history of heavy alcohol intake, hypothyroidism, steroid intake, or other conditions.

The patient's acute medical condition often compromises both the mental status and the examination itself. A patient in acute pain cannot be expected to give full attention to the subtraction of sevens or to remembering three objects in the here and now or events in the distant past. The removal of dentures may make it difficult for the patient to articulate. The interviewer can only get as much data as possible under the circumstances and register and record both the data and the circumstances. All information is of potential value.

Physical Examination

The performance of physical examinations is another subject about which psychiatrists differ. Some feel that physical interaction with a patient, beyond that of polite social interaction (shaking hands, a pat on the back or arm), can provoke confounding emotional reactions in the psychiatrist-patient relationship. Others stress the importance of making some physical contact with the patient (Yager 1989). A psychiatrist not in the habit of physically examining patients may feel that his or her skills are no longer adequate. However, the procedures relevant to a psychiatric consultation tend to be well within the average psychiatrist's capacity. And drawing on the skills and training psychiatrists have as physicians solidifies their identity as physicians in the eyes of other hospital staff, consultees, and patients.

Transference and countertransference issues are different in the context of a busy, open hospital floor than in the isolation of a private office. Paying attention to the somatic concerns that occasioned the hospitalization and cause distress to the patient reinforces the idea that the psychiatrist is genuinely interested and helpful, and a physician, as well. On the other hand, many consultants are successful and appreciated even though they limit physical contact with patients to handshakes.

It is not only empathic but informative to take a look at areas of the patient's body that are hurting and/or diseased. Occasionally, the consultant discovers a physical finding that has been overlooked. In other cases, one's comprehension of the patient's feelings of disfigurement, exhaustion, or mistreatment is increased by the sight of physical lesions. The antecubital area completely bruised by attempted and infected phlebotomies gives an impression that helps the consultant understand a patient's difficulty in seeing the staff as helpful and in consenting to further interventions.

The consultant may choose to perform components of a neurological examination. This is another procedure that is often performed cursorily, if at all, on nonneurological services. The patient's difficulty with vision, coordination, hearing, locomotion, or sensation, for example, may well be a significant element of the condition for which consultation has been sought. Competence at basic neurological evaluation identifies the psychiatric consultant as a doctor of the CNS. The very sight of a psychiatrist with tools of the medical trade can change the antiquated attitudes of other medical specialists and other psychiatrists and is an effective model for medical students and residents in psychiatry.

Vital signs can be assessed by anyone with minimum training and are essential to the diagnosis of conditions leading to organic brain syndromes, drug overdoses or abuse, and complications of psychoactive agents. Transient hypotensive episodes may explain the patient's passing confusional states. Finally, the observation and recording of the patient's general physical condition are major factors in many consultations. Wasting may be a clue to depression or to dementia interfering with the patient's capacity to obtain nourishment. A very poor overall condition may be an indication of a hopeless lesion or terminal situation that the patient suspects, but that the staff has not discussed with the patient. This may be the source of the "rule out depression" that was the stated reason for the referral. A patient who is extremely fit probably has a lot of investment in physical well-being and may adapt poorly to a condition or intervention that limits physical mobility.

OBSERVING THE ENVIRONMENT

Pay attention to the objects and persons in the patient's environment and their interaction. A patient who is usually mildly demented may be utterly confused in a multibed ward filled with noisy visitors, televisions, medical equipment, and so forth. A patient's depressive symptoms may be exacerbated by a hospital environment lacking in stimulation. The patient may brighten, or become visibly upset, when a certain person enters or leaves the room. A profusion of floral arrangements and boxes of candy tells the consultant that there is some sort of social network, while a total reliance on hospital-issue garments and supplies bespeaks the opposite.

Sometimes the environment is the crux of the problem. For example, one of the authors was called emergently to see a man in his forties who had been admitted to the medical unit for the treatment of delirium tremens. Despite the administration of large doses of benzodiazepines, the patient had broken through three sets of leather wrist and ankle restraints and was threatening to the staff and quite possibly dangerous to himself. At the door of the patient's room, the consultant stopped to assess the situation. Broken leather straps and overturned pitchers lay around a newly re-restrained, strong, vigorous man who was making every effort to free himself, thrashing and shouting.

Every so often, momentarily exhausted, he stopped and lay still and quiet. During these intervals, the nurse assigned to sit constantly with and monitor him was observed to say, "Are you going to be good now? If you are, you can have a drag on my cigarette." She moved the cigarette toward his lips and then jerked it abruptly away, taunting, "Are you sure you're going to be good?" Then the patient would roar and strain in frustration and rage. The consultant arranged for this nurse to be replaced immediately by someone more calming; the patient fell asleep without any additional medication or intervention, slept soundly for 18 hours, and woke calm and cooperative.

In another case, a patient whose consultation request read "paranoid" was in a hospital room next to the nursing station, where he could actually see and hear, as could the consultant, members of the staff discussing his case and laughing about his complaints, personality, intellect, and family. The patient was indeed chronically suspicious, pessimistic, and isolated. But in both of these real and typical cases, the patient's diagnosis had led to stigmatization, dehumanization, and poor care. The patients' reactive rage was understandable. Not only the psychiatrists' suggested changes in management but the very validation of the patients' perception by the psychiatrists is humanizing and healing.

Conveying Preliminary Impressions to the Patient

Although the consultant may feel that further observation, tests, or history is necessary before a firm diagnosis can be made, some communication should be made to the patient before leaving the bedside. Sum up the data you have gathered in language the patient can understand. This gives the patient an opportunity to correct or amplify it. Express your empathy for the patient's suffering. Tell the patient what additional material you think you will need and how you plan to obtain it: "Perhaps your spouse can bring in those nerve pills you were taking." "I want to see how your thinking clears up as you recover from the operation."

Discuss with the patient, again in appropriate terms, the psychodynamics that appear to be significant. ("I think your chest pain frightened and depressed you because you think you will die of a heart attack at an early age, like your father. But your condition is different, and medical care has improved. Your doctors think you have an excellent chance of recovery.") Not infrequently, a single diagnostic interview stimulates the patient's introspection: "You're absolutely right; my arthritis always hurts more after I have a fight with my daughter-in-law. I'd like to smack her, but I guess I'd be better off doing the exercises the doctor recommended." Many patients can work independently on the insight gained and change their interactions with their significant others, or their reactions to the stress of illness (Blacher 1984).

If you have a reasonably firm and possibly helpful working diagnosis and prognosis, share them with the patient. A label alone is not helpful, but the knowledge that one has a specific, treatable, or self-limited disease may be. Explain how you have arrived at your conclusion: "Your difficulties with sleep, appetite, concentration, pleasure, and mood indicate that you are suffering from a depression. This is a significant, but common and treatable, condition. There is an excellent chance you will respond to medication and psychotherapy." "I think you have been confused because your blood sugar was so low. Your thinking will probably clear up now." Doctors tend to be overly pessimistic. If we predict the worst, we come out as either excellent diagnosticians or miracle workers. But recovery is sometimes, and improvement often, and hope always, reasonable to suggest. Your optimism is tremendously important to the patient.

Tell the patient your immediate plans. You will discuss your findings with the primary physician; negotiate about specifics of the history that the patient would prefer you withheld. You may intend to contact the social worker and solicit help locating or working with the family, or straightening out the patient's public aid or social security status. Perhaps you think it would be a good idea to extend the visiting hours or change the visiting rules for this patient so as to allow contact with a spouse with an odd work schedule or to set the patient's mind at rest about his or her children. If you are reasonably sure that your advice will be followed, inform the patient that you will be recommending that a psycho-active medication be prescribed or that medication in use be decreased or discontinued. Otherwise, wait until you have spoken to the primary physician so as not to confuse the patient.

Finally, solicit the patient's reaction to the interview as a whole: "How did it feel to talk about these things with me?" This question demonstrates respect for the patient's viewpoint and is an indicator of the patient's likely response to psychotherapy. Ask whether the patient has any questions. Inform the patient when you intend to return, how long you will spend, and what you will next do together with the patient (MacKinnon and Michels 1971).

REFERENCES

American Psychiatric Association: The Principles of Medical Ethics, With Annotations Especially Applicable to Psychiatry. Washington, DC, American Psychiatric Association, 1985

Bellak L, Small L: Emergency Psychotherapy and Brief Psychotherapy. New York, Grune & Stratton, 1965

Blacher RS: The briefest encounter: psychotherapy for medical and surgical patients. Gen Hosp Psychiatry 6:226–232, 1984

Colon EA, Popkin M, Callies A: Emergency psychiatric consultation to medical-surgical services. Psychosomatics 29:3–10, 1988

Dvoredsky AE, Cooley HW: Comparative severity of illness in patients with combined medical and psychiatric diagnoses. Psychosomatics 27:625–630, 1986

Finkel JB: The medical interview and the therapeutic alliance, in Psychiatric Management for Medical Practitioners. Edited by Kornfeld DS, Finkel JB. New York, Grune & Stratton, 1982, pp 1–18

Garrick TR, Stotland NL: How to write a psychiatric consultation. Am J Psychiatry 139:849–855, 1982

Glazer WM, Astrachan BM: Social systems approach to consultation-liaison psychiatry. Int J Psychiatry Med 9:33–47, 1978–1979

Groves JE: Management of the borderline patient on a medical or surgical ward: the psychiatric consultant's role. Int J Psychiatry Med 6:337–348, 1975

Illinois, General Assembly: Mental Health and Developmental Disabilities Confidentiality Act, PA80-1508, 1988

Kahana RJ, Bibring GL: Personality types in medical management, in Psychiatry and Medical Practice in a General Hospital. Edited by Zinberg N. New York, International Universities Press, 1964, pp 108–123

Kahn RL: Brief objective measures for the determination of mental status in the aged. Am J Psychiatry 117:326–328, 1960

Kimball CP: Techniques of interviewing. I. Interviewing and the meaning of the symptom. Ann Intern Med 71:147–153, 1969

Kimball CP: The Biopsychosocial Approach to the Patient. Baltimore, MD, Williams & Wilkins, 1981

Koran LM, Van Natta J, Stephens JR, et al: Patients' reactions to psychiatric consultation. JAMA 241:1603–1605, 1979

Lipowski ZJ: Review of consultation psychiatry and psychosomatic medicine. II. Clinical aspects. Psychosom Med 19:201–224, 1967

MacKinnon RA, Michels R: The Psychiatric Interview in Clinical Practice. Philadelphia, PA, WB Saunders, 1971

Meyer E, Mendelson M: Psychiatric consultations with patients on medical and surgical wards. Psychiatry 24:197–220, 1961

Mills MJ, Daniels ML: Medical-legal issues, in Principles of Medical Psychiatry. Edited by Stoudemire MD, Fogel BS. Orlando, FL, Grune & Stratton, 1987, pp 463–476

Murray GB: Confusion, delirium, and dementia, in Massachusetts General Hospital Handbook of General Hospital Psychiatry, 2nd Edition. Edited by Hackett TP, Cassem NH. Littleton, MA, PSG Publishers, 1987, pp 84–115

Rogers RR, Rasof B: The gap between psychiatric practice and the medical model. Compr Psychiatry 9:459–463, 1977

Strain JJ: Psychological reactions to medical illness and hospitalization, in Psychological Care of the Medically Ill. Edited by Strain JJ, Grossman S. New York, Appleton-Century-Crofts, 1975, pp 11–22

Weisman AD: Coping with illness, in Massachusetts General Hospital Handbook of General Hospital Psychiatry, 2nd Edition. Edited by Hackett TP, Cassem NH. Littleton, MA, PSG Publishers, 1987, pp 297–308

Yager J: Specific components of bedside manner in the general hospital psychiatric consultation: twelve concrete suggestions. Psychosomatics 30:209–212, 1989

7

What to Do Before Leaving the Medical Unit

After leaving the patient's bedside, the consultant often writes a note and leaves to pursue other activities. But there are a number of interventions that are optimally considered and attended to before leaving the medical unit. First is the pursuit of further information. Whether or not the consultant has reviewed the patient's chart and discussed the case with the medical, nursing, and ancillary staffs and the patient's family before interviewing the patient, the interval of time and the contact with the patient may refocus the consultant's attention and/or make gaps in the information apparent.

Administrative and legal issues may require action. The consultant may find it necessary to make urgent recommendations that must be brought to the staff's attention before the written consultation is seen, and acted upon, by the responsible physician. Medical and nursing staff members are sometimes waiting for and/or responsive to the consultant's immediate observations.

While some of these problems can be addressed by telephone from the consultant's office or other location, there are advantages to accomplishing them before leaving the hospital floor. The chart, the names, and the phone or pager numbers of others to whom the consultant needs to speak, as well as other information, are more available. The continued presence of the consultant makes the urgency of the need to obtain information, or carry out immediate recommendations, more compelling.

ANOTHER LOOK AT THE AVAILABLE INFORMATION

The Chart

The encounter with the patient clarifies diagnostic and therapeutic questions posed by the primary physician and the other questions preliminarily conceptualized by the consultant. These now-focused questions give rise to a need for specific items of information. Some answers may be found in the hospital chart. For example, although the referral made no reference to this problem, you discover that the patient has signs and symptoms of an organic brain syndrome. You go back to the chart to look more carefully for indications of CNS infection, drug toxicity, etc. You search for notations about the patient's mental status before, at, and/or since admission (Slaby and Cullen 1987).

Perhaps you have arrived at the bedside to find the patient somnolent and groggy, difficult to engage in dialogue. Her breathing appears labored. You now need to know what analgesics and narcotics are being administered, and in what doses. When was the last dose given? Do the blood gases indicate hypoxemia? Do laboratory values suggest renal or hepatic failure? Do the nursing notes indicate that the patient has previously been more alert—perhaps chatted with the nurses, other staff, or visitors—at other times?

The Staff

On these or related subjects, you may want to obtain further information from staff present on the unit. If you have had trouble getting the patient to offer information, you may be particularly interested in finding someone skilled at getting the patient to talk. Sometimes, for example, a patient whose native tongue is not English—who either has not mastered English or has difficulty communicating in English under the stress of illness—gives up trying to explain symptoms or get help and withdraws from contact with the staff. He seems to be depressed, schizoid, hostile, and/or suspicious. The patient may appear entirely different—animated and related—with a family or staff member who speaks his native language. If the patient has no friends or family present, it is often worthwhile to seek a translator somewhere in the hospital community. More than once, we and a patient have been helped a great deal by a secretary or hospital engineer fluent in a language unusual in our geographic area. Although access and timing may be difficult, it is our experience that the unofficial translator is very gratified to perform this service.

Once in a while the consultant's inquiry about recent mental status changes precipitates a discovery crucial to the patient's diagnosis and treatment. In one case, consultation was sought because of a patient's decrease in speech, which was thought to be due to depression. The consultant found that the patient was having difficulty finding the words to express thoughts; after the interview, he asked the staff. The nurses stated that no problem had been noticed in the preceding days. The expressive aphasia, then worked up, turned out to be a symptom of a small stroke secondary to carotid atherosclerosis, which was then effectively treated. In another case, the onset of a patient's massively decreased activity and speech was traced to the time he learned of a death of another patient with a similar illness, whom he had met, befriended, and followed on the hospital ward. Brief psychodynamic therapy addressing this dynamic was indicated and carried out, with successful results.

Sometimes the consultant's observations do not agree with those of the staff. This is equally important to address after the patient interview. For example, consultation is sought because the patient is "paranoid." The consultant finds an intellectually slow patient, angry and suspicious because she has suffered a succession of complications from what was expected to be straightforward surgery (Yager 1975). There is no evidence of psychotic ideation. Inquiring of the nurse what made the staff concerned that the patient was paranoid, the consultant is told that she said, "No one here cares what happens to me. They just hurt me."

Discrepancy between the consultant's observations and those of the staff may be a clue to borderline or other character psychopathology (Groves 1987), or to an unresolved psychiatric emergency. Perhaps the patient does behave as though deeply depressed in some company and under some circumstances, but not in others. He or she may seem like "an entirely different person" with some members of the staff than with others. The patient who has committed a crime, and is hoping for judicial leniency based on psychiatric impairment, may sound bizarre only in the presence of the primary physician, consultant, and police. A suicidal patient may confess self-destructive thoughts or intentions to staff or family, but deny them to the psychiatric consultant because of fear of involuntary psychiatric hospitalization (Davidson 1987). These sorts of discrepancies call for clarification after the interview (Kimball 1977).

It is also important to corroborate with the staff the patient's communications about diagnosis, prognosis, and treatment plan. Has the patient misunderstood or overreacted? Has the staff neglected to explain, or does the patient have trouble registering information despite repeated accounts (Yager 1975)? If the despondent patient has incorrectly understood someone to say that his or her case is hopeless, it may be important to trace the source so that the same person can correct the misapprehension. Or the consultant may simply want to corroborate the information so as to help the patient face whatever outcome or intervention is logically anticipated.

The account of a particular sequence of events may be at issue. It may be that the patient needs a staff member to explain exactly what happened during the time he or she was delirious. Or the consultant may need to elicit the staff's impression of an event that the patient experienced as terrifying, cruel, or neglectful. Was the unit indeed short-staffed, or does this particular patient ring the nurses' bell so frequently that it is impossible or unrewarding to try to respond? Were there multiple unsuccessful attempts at venipuncture, lumbar puncture, placement of a central venous line? Does a particular doctor indeed come across as arrogant, uncaring, or even cruel? The psychiatrist's job is to take the patient's account seriously, but neutrally (Kahana 1964). Disturbing material must prompt careful investigation.

Family and Friends

The case of an elderly man who had suffered a stroke was discussed earlier (see Chapter 5) as an example of the importance of information obtained from family and friends; a description of his premorbid personality and attitude toward handicaps by a friend who chanced on the scene after a consultation interview was a major factor in the diagnosis of depression. Most of the issues are similar to those discussed above with regard to the staff. While the staff is more equipped to make objective and expert observations of the patient's recent behavior, family and friends have much more information about baseline and premorbid mental status, and changes in this status. Because this information may be gathered earlier in the consultation, much of this material has been presented in previous chapters. However, the request for consultation and preliminary contacts with the physician and staff may give no hint that this information will be crucial to diagnosis and treatment. Therefore, the consultant will seek it actively for the first time after the interview.

People who have known the patient for some time can offer valuable insights into the dynamics of the patient's personality and typical responses to illness (Strain and Grossman 1975). Was there a psychosocial stress that preceded the onset of symptoms? How does the patient usually respond to physical illness? Has he or she ever had the same or similar symptoms and signs before? Have other family members? What do family members think is the appropriate diagnosis?—workup?—treatment? Are they satisfied with the care the patient is getting, the information they are receiving, and the practical visiting arrangements, such as visiting hours and sleeping accommodations? Do they communicate suspicion and discontent to the patient, absorb the patient's complaints, or mediate helpfully between patient and hospital unit?

What is the baseline social situation? Does the patient live alone and care for himself or herself? Are grown children close, involved, and available; intrusive; or long or recently absent? Is the care of the patient's young children a concern (Milano 1982)? Have the children been left in circumstances with which the patient does not feel comfortable? Is the family at a loss as to how to tell the children about the illness or handle their visiting the patient?

How are significant others reacting to the illness and hospitalization? A patient may be deeply disappointed by what he or she perceives to be a lack of concern, worried about the drain on loving and supportive family members, or frantic because they are frantic. Not infrequently, significant others of patients requiring psychiatric consultation feel "at the end of their rope" with the patient and the illness. Now that you have seen the patient, you may be more empathic with their frustration and exhaustion—or curious about their resources and attitudes. Plans for discharge are often critical to the patient's mood. Has the family communicated a disinclination to take the patient home from the hospital, or an intention to move the patient from an independent living situation to a nursing facility or the home of a relative? The patient will sense and react to such ideas whether they are verbally stated or not (Strain 1978).

Interviewing the patient's family and friends after the interview with the patient raises issues of confidentiality (Engelhardt and McCullough 1979). This issue resurfaces at this point in the process because significant others may well be waiting to hear the consultant's opinion after the examination of the patient. And the consultant is often tempted to convey the information obtained to those most interested in the patient's welfare. The consultant can listen to anything, but he or she cannot tell anyone about the patient's condition without the patient's permission. Even the fact that a psychiatrist has been consulted may be privileged. If necessary, go back to the bedside and negotiate with the patient about the necessity for, and limits on, communication with others. There are exceptions to the patient's privilege, such as the duty to warn (Stone 1984). Such a case arises when a patient admitted for injuries threatens to retaliate against the perpetrator. If, in your expert opinion, the patient may be a significant risk of some kind, and significant others are loathe to communicate important information, you may choose to violate confidentiality and disclose something of the danger so as to elicit their cooperation. For example, knowledge of a history of illegal or prescription drug abuse is often central to effective care (Renner 1987). There are also circumstances in which you may tell the family that there is something important that the patient has forbidden you to tell anyone, and leave them to negotiate with the patient.

THE NEED FOR OUTSIDE INFORMATION

Past Medical Records

There are occasions when the current chart and available informants leave significant gaps in the history. When the consultation reveals a past history of psychiatric illness and treatment, the records from former hospitalizations or outpatient interventions may be urgently required. Knowledge of past diagnostic procedures and successful and unsuccessful psychopharmacologic regimens can forestall unnecessary duplication and frustration for staff, and suffering for the patient. It is also important to know when the patient has been hospitalized many times, and undergone countless diagnostic procedures and invasive maneuvers for similar symptoms, to no avail.

Notes regarding suspicion that the illness is factitious, as well as corroborative evidence, may be buried in the old records. These records may contain information about guardianship, next of kin, and baseline mental status. In order to facilitate effective management, the consultant may well want to set a search for these records in motion before leaving the unit.

Other Sources

Psychiatric consultation may reveal the need for other kinds of information as well. The possibility that the patient has a guardian was just mentioned. Other kinds of judicial proceedings may have been completed or may be under way. The patient may be in the process of suing someone he claims injured him, or a former physician and/or hospital. When the interview gives clues to these circumstances, the consultant will want to know whether the consultation, and the consultant, may become part of a court proceeding. Was the patient uncooperative with the consultation because the suspicion of psychiatric illness may cast doubt on the reliability of his testimony? Or does the patient hope that the psychiatrist will testify that he has suffered grievous emotional damage?

Psychiatrists who do not deal regularly with forensic issues, and nonpsychiatric staff, may have a low index of suspicion for sociopathic behavior and character. Again, the interview might yield the first evidence that this may be the case. The patient may have been accused, or found guilty, of civil or criminal misconduct. This fact could be crucial in management. Other patients and staff may need to be protected. A search of belongings, confinement to a single room, and/or assignment of a security guard may be necessary. Transfer to a hospital that is part of the criminal justice system could be considered. The patient may be likely to obtain, use, and/or distribute substances of abuse during the hospitalization. Or the patient may be using the fact of hospitalization, or medical or psychiatric symptoms, to avoid punishment. Concern about any of these possibilities may lead the consultant to initiate a search for legal documents before leaving the floor.

The consultant may wish to obtain information about resources and constraints applicable to this particular case. For example, would it be possible to transfer an overstimulated or paranoid patient to a private room? Is a 24-hour "sitter," "one-to-one," or monitor available? Could arrangements be made to allow a competent and reassuring relative to remain with the patient at all times, or at certain problematic times such as overnight or during upsetting medical procedures? Is there insurance coverage for psychiatric hospitalization or outpatient care? Is there a bed available in the hospital's, or another appropriate, psychiatric unit? Initiating the search for all these kinds of information may be most practical while the consultant is still on the unit, where insurance numbers, hospital unit numbers, and other data about the patient and the system are more available than they will be in the psychiatrist's office.

Finally, the chart or the staff may indicate that important tests have been ordered or performed. If the results are not in the chart, the consultant can call, or request that staff call, the laboratories and/or radiology or pathology department to see whether findings are available. For example, the consultant may infer from the interview that a patient awaiting biopsy results may decompensate if informed he or she has a malignancy. It is obviously optimal to have all possible data registered, assimilated, and acted upon before leaving the scene, and before contacting the primary physician to discuss the case. It is also another demonstration of expertise and commitment.

ADMINISTRATIVE AND LEGAL ISSUES

Many of these issues have been covered in the foregoing section, because they have to do with interactions with the patient, significant others, or staff. We can summarize them here. The presence of the consultant on the hospital floor underscores the seriousness of the psychiatric problem and the consultant's clinical involvement and availability. Meeting with other personnel on, or making calls from, the hospital floor sets their involvement in motion, makes potential problems or obstacles manifest, and allows the consultant to make notations in the chart about the results of these interactions—with health-care professionals, with the hospital administration, or with the legal department or consultant.

When a need for collaboration with, or referral to, the social worker or social work department, or any other allied professional, has been identified, the consultant can telephone from the unit to discuss the case and reach an agreement about respective roles, responsibilities, and schedules. Calling to share clinical impressions and problems, rather than leaving a recommendation in the chart (e.g., "Social worker to arrange for nursing home placement"), gives a meaningful message that the psychiatrist respects and values other professionals' opinions and contributions.

This process fosters interdisciplinary trust and cooperation. The social worker may suggest psychiatric consultation for the next case on the unit. The consultant will be forewarned should there be some problem with the referral, such as a vacation or overloaded schedule. And the other professional will have the opportunity to inform the consultant, should he or she already have garnered information and begun an intervention not yet entered in the chart.

In cases in which current or potential administrative and/or medicolegal problems are identified, the consultant may want to call the appropriate hospital department from the unit. There is nothing quite so compelling as a call beginning, "I am calling from the X Unit, where I have just seen Ms. S.," or "I will wait with Ms. S. until you set a guardianship procedure in motion— obtain bars for the windows—find a way to order a 24-hour sitter for the patient." Situations such as those alluded to here raise difficult, core questions about psychiatric consultation. Should the psychiatrist volunteer to provide this type of intervention or protection? It is unlikely to be financially compensated. On the other hand, can the consultant be (and seem) a responsible physician without making such interventions at times? Can a physician leave the scene when a patient is hemorrhaging or choking—or suicidal—before the patient's safety is assured? Establishing workable, professional limits and managing time are particular challenges in the consultation setting.

Typical situations are (a) questions about the ability to give "good" consent for treatment, (b) the need for guardianship or commitment, (c) the patient's wish to leave against medical advice, (d) a difference of opinion among close relatives as to how a patient whose own judgment is compromised ought to be treated, (e) difficulty obtaining appropriate staffing or physical circumstances to keep the patient and others safe, and (f) the litigious and threatening patient (Mills and Daniels 1987). Should the administrator or lawyer have questions, the floor staff, chart, patient, and patient's family are nearby resources. You can make sure your name, phone number, and available times are clearly understood so that you can be reached for further discussion.

URGENT RECOMMENDATIONS

All recommendations are entered in the chart as part of the written consultation. Some consultants dictate this document and send or deliver it to the chart or referring physician hours or days after the consultation is performed. Others, as we recommend, write it immediately. However, the consultant has no way of knowing when it will be read by the physicians responsible for the patient, and then when or whether the suggestions will be implemented. The consultant will at times, like those indicated above, identify needs that are urgent. Personal, immediate communication underscores their urgency and increases the likelihood that the relevant recommendations will be carried out.

Consultants are, by definition, not primary physicians, but psychiatrists are primary physicians in other contexts. As primary physicians, we deal with life-and-death matters and take responsibility for patients' health and safety. Perhaps this aspect of our functioning is not always appreciated by nonpsychiatrists. So attention to urgent recommendations serves both to address the needs of the individual patient and to reinforce the concept of psychiatry as a practical, vital discipline. There are several categories of urgent recommendations.

As mentioned above, the psychiatric consultant may arrive at the bedside to discover the patient in an acute state of medical deterioration. What was thought to be "rule out depression" turns out to be terminal deficits in respiratory, cardiac, and/or CNS function, or partially suppressed status epilepticus and postictal changes. The patient's confusion may be secondary to life-threatening metabolic imbalance. The patient's aberrant behavior may be precipitated by a space-occupying (and expanding) brain lesion. If any of these conditions, or others, are immediately threatening to the patient's health or life, the consultant cannot leave the unit without making sure that a member of the primary team has been notified and has assumed responsibility for the situation.

Related situations are those in which a "psychiatric" condition or complication demands urgent medical intervention. The patient's psychosis may be a sign of drug toxicity, withdrawal, or overdose. The consultant may have diagnosed neuroleptic malignant syndrome or water intoxication. A paranoid patient may be refusing vital oral medications, nourishment, or fluids.

The urgent problem may be a different sort of behavioral dangerousness, posing external bodily risk to the patient. These are cases in which some sort of physical limitation to the patient's freedom must be considered and seen to. The patient may simply need the guard rails to be kept up on the side of the bed at all times. This kind of treatment can serve to remind a somewhat confused patient to stay in bed or obtain assistance with ambulation, prevent a delirious and agitated patient from falling out of bed, or suggest a physical protection, like an infant's crib, to a regressed and anxious patient.

More confining physical restraints may be necessary to prevent the patient from hurting himself or herself, or others. Some state mental-health codes, hospital regulations, and procedural manuals outline guidelines for the use of restraints. The consultant must be familiar with regulations in his or her geographic area and treatment setting. A patient whose mental state has impaired the capacity to act in his or her own best interest may urgently need a guardian to make decisions.

When the danger is that the patient will leave the hospital unit, both without being capable of weighing the risks and making an informed decision, and at immediate risk to safety, a variety of deterrents may be set in place. The patient can be committed, either to the medical or the psychiatric unit. Again, laws and regulations vary from location to location (Groves and Vaccarino

120   Manual of Psychiatric Consultation

1987). The nursing staff and hospital security guards may simply
be alerted to watch for the patient and gently return him or her to
bed. Physical restraints can be used. And when elopement or
immediate physical danger is at issue, one-to-one, 24-hour surveillance by a staff member, or, under certain circumstances, a
relative, may be decided upon.

In the author's experience, the use of such "sitters," as they are
often called, is many times initiated without careful delineation
and realistic consideration of goals, responsibilities, and capabili-
ties. A sitter may be conceptualized as simply a calm, objective,
and caring human being who reassures the patient by being present, by offering orienting cues, and by keeping a general watch
on the patient's behavior. At times, however, a sitter seems to be
expected to be a kind of expert on psychiatric management, keeping an intense, professional surveillance on the patient's signs
and symptoms, and offering some form of supportive psychotherapy as clinically indicated. A one-to-one nurse on a psychiatric unit, for example, would be expected to make expert observations and notations about the progress of the patient's psychiatric
disorder, such as behavior suggestive of hallucinatory experiences. Such a nurse would make focused, thoughtful, and effective verbal interventions—for example, to encourage a patient to
wonder about the meanings of his or her behavior or try to
remember relevant past events; to offer suggestions about reducing anxiety or dealing with troublesome family members.

A major problem is the implicit expectation that a sitter will
physically prevent the patient from leaving or inflicting damage
on self or others. Sitters available in many nonpsychiatric medical
settings are neither psychologically nor physically capable of
carrying out this expectation. The consultant may return to find
an agitated, threatening man who is large and muscular being
monitored by an elderly, frail woman attendant.

Depending on the institution and the situation, family members may be encouraged, allowed, or forbidden to serve as constant companions or monitors for patients. The issues in all these
situations are the same as with paid staff, and, especially when
the sitter is ordered on the advice of the psychiatric consultant, it
is up to the consultant to address them. Is there agreement
between the hospital and the proposed sitter about what service
is to be provided? Is the sitter capable of providing it? In addition

to the considerations of physical strength, the question of constant surveillance and attendance is more difficult than it might seem.

Like sterile technique in the surgical suite, one-to-one monitoring is a set of behaviors that requires theoretical understanding, preparation, and practice. Keeping a patient in constant view is a necessity difficult for those other than experienced psychiatric experts to conceptualize and fulfill. We have often observed that staff or relatives accepting an assignment to stay with the patient nevertheless leave to go to the bathroom, make a telephone call, eat, or "allow the patient some privacy to visit with friends or go to the toilet," without realizing that these absences pose a danger.

The consultant has to make the purpose of the recommendation for the sitter clear, indicate what is expected, and communicate the orders directly to the proposed attendant at times. Clinical examples of moments of inattention leading to tragic consequences may drive the point home. Insist that the attendant note, verbatim, problematic verbal and behavioral communications of the patient. Discuss how the attendant should respond to psychotic or otherwise difficult statements. The consultant may also be involved in the decision as to whether a particular staff or family member is suitable for the task. One person may be reassuring, while another is an irritant.

Recommendations may be urgent even in the absence of immediate physical danger. There are often elements of the patient's hospital environment that are unnecessarily irritating, disturbing, and/or painful. It may be the patient's roommate(s), or a roommate's guests, whose behavior or mere presence keeps the patient from resting, exacerbating sleep deprivation, rage, and confusion. A particular staff member may be unable to get along with the patient, so that the patient is anxious, aroused, or furious at both the reality and the prospect of interactions with that person. The patient may have been observed to decompensate during or after visits from certain individuals. If any of these situations is significantly contributing to the patient's psychiatric symptoms, the consultant may want to see that changes are arranged before leaving the unit. If the problematic situation is occurring at the time of the consultation, the consultant can use that opportunity to allow the staff to observe it.

SHARING FIRST IMPRESSIONS

A variety of situations in which it is advisable to discuss diagnostic and management issues with members of the nursing and/or medical staff before leaving the unit have been described in this chapter. These are conditions that require the urgent search for more information or institution of interventions to prevent danger to the patient or others. The consultant's continuing physical presence on the unit underscores the importance of the matter at hand. But it is also a good idea to discuss every case with the available staff before departing. Although the consultant will enter a written note into the chart, there is nothing that has an impact like the personal presence of the consultant (Hengeveld and Rooymans 1983). Even if the patient was not available on the floor, or was not able to communicate for some reason, the fact that the consultant has attempted to provide service means a great deal (De-Nour 1978).

If the preliminary gathering of information and formulation have been completed, verbal communication reinforces assimilation of the proffered advice. Personal contact enables the consultant to evaluate the response of the consultee, adapting language, tone, and content as the dialogue proceeds (Popkin and Mackenzie 1984). In addition to facilitating the care of the patient, the psychiatrist can identify educational needs to address in consultations and formal educational exercises in the future (Martin 1975).

The psychiatrist's observations, questions, and suggestions often stimulate the consultee to remember relevant material. The consultant can attempt to reconcile conflicts among information obtained from the chart, the patient, and other sources. It will also be possible to determine what kinds of recommendations are acceptable and feasible. It may become apparent that some simply do not appeal to the consultee; for example, the internist is simply not willing to try a tricyclic antidepressant in a patient with a cardiac lesion, despite scientific studies demonstrating its safety in cases similar to the patient's. If immediate negotiation and education fail, the consultant will be aware and can begin to consider alternative persuasive and/or treatment approaches. Other suggestions will raise practical, rather than medical, problems: for example, the unavailability of sitters on a particular nursing shift or of private rooms on a particular service.

In these and some other cases, a discussion preceding the written consultation can prevent the entry of problematic notations in the chart. For example, the consultant may think it advisable that the patient remain in the general hospital for further observation and treatment. However, if the utilization review committee, the insurance company, or other outside forces present obstacles to this course, it may be preferable to work out an acceptable compromise by collegial discussion. A written, adversarial debate in the patient's chart may put the primary service, the hospital, and even the consultant at legal risk and alienate them from each other and from psychiatry.

Situations of this kind commonly occur around competence and discharge planning. The consultant must bear in mind the fact that the indications for therapeutic and legal decisions are seldom absolute. A patient who was groggy or frightened during the psychiatric interview may have a long history of clearly expressed intentions about his or her care, which is well known to the primary physician and/or family. A patient who would be unable to care for himself or herself in a strange or isolated setting, or in the hospital, may be very well cared for by relatives at home or may be able to manage adequately in a familiar environment. In face-to-face discussion, you might convince the service to postpone discharge and/or obtain information that makes discharge a more tenable plan. Do not enter conclusions about guardianship, discharge, or competence in the chart until you have had a chance to discuss them.

A patient's medical condition may temporarily compromise mental status and judgment. This situation is so common in the general hospital that if each case were adjudicated, both the medical and the judicial systems would likely be overwhelmed. It is impossible and unnecessary to declare legally incompetent every patient who is under anesthesia, in the recovery room, in shock, toxic, highly febrile, etc. The unconsidered notation that the patient is unable to give "good" consent may delay diagnosis and treatment and thereby compromise care. A combination of psychiatric expertise, ethics, sophistication, and common sense is required.

The consultant may also wish to communicate verbally information that, while not strictly confidential, might best be kept out of the chart (Engelhardt and McCullough 1979). The fact that the patient is upset because a relative was accused or convicted of a criminal offense, or that a divorce is pending, can make the patient's behavior comprehensible and therefore tolerable to the primary-care team. It need not be available to the insurance carrier, employer, and everyone else who has access to the medical record. The sensitive information may relate to the hospital, rather than the patient; a behavioral problem may be associated with the care of a particular nurse, who seems otherwise competent and caring, or with a mistake or miscommunication. Maligning members of the staff in a legal document such as the chart will not help the patient in most cases and will surely undermine the relationship between the consultant and staff members.

It is up to each consultant to filter information to enter into the written record, weighing medicolegal, ethical, and clinical factors. His or her presence on the clinical unit to discuss findings makes manifest psychiatric participation in the work going on there—psychiatric responsiveness, psychiatric thoroughness in information seeking, psychiatric concern about the patient's well-being, and psychiatric availability for discussion. It may prevent interruptions in ensuing activities and the need to spend time trying to reach staff or family members later, and increase the likelihood of other consultations. One of the most common complaints of dissatisfied former, current, or potential consultees is, "I never see that psychiatrist on my service."

REFERENCES

Davidson L: Suicide and violence in the medical setting, in Principles of Medical Psychiatry. Edited by Stoudemire MC, Fogel BS. Orlando, FL, Grune & Stratton, 1987, pp 237–252

De-Nour AK: Attitudes of physicians in a general hospital towards a psychiatric consultation service. Mental Health and Society 5:215–223, 1978

Engelhardt HT Jr, McCullough LB: Confidentiality in the consultation-liaison process. Psychiatr Clin North Am 2:403–413, 1979

Groves JE: Borderline patients, in Massachusetts General Hospital Handbook of General Hospital Psychiatry, 2nd Edition. Edited by Hackett TP, Cassem NH. Littleton, MA, PSG Publishers, 1987, pp 184–207

Groves JE, Vaccarino JM: Legal aspects of consultation, in Massachusetts General Hospital Handbook of General Hospital Psychiatry, 2nd Edition. Edited by Hackett TP, Cassem NH. Littleton, MA, PSG Publishers, 1987, pp 591–617

Hengeveld MW, Rooymans HGM: The relevance of a staff-oriented approach in consultation psychiatry: a preliminary study. Gen Hosp Psychiatry 5:259–264, 1983

Kahana RJ: Teaching medical psychology through psychiatric consultation, in Psychiatry and Medical Practice in a General Hospital. Edited by Zinberg NE. New York, International Universities Press, 1964, pp 98–107

Kimball CP: The languages of psychosomatic medicine. Psychother Psychosom 28:1–12, 1977

Martin LR: Liaison psychiatry and the education of the family practitioner, in Consultation-Liaison Psychiatry. Edited by Pasnau RO. New York, Grune & Stratton, 1975, pp 285–294

Milano MR: The management of family and marital problems, in Psychiatric Management for Medical Practitioners. Edited by Kornfeld DS, Finkel JB. New York, Grune & Stratton, 1982, pp 168–184

Mills MJ, Daniels ML: Medical-legal issues, in Principles of Medical Psychiatry. Edited by Stoudemire MD, Fogel BS. Orlando, FL, Grune & Stratton, 1987, pp 463–476

Popkin MD, Mackenzie TB: Communicating with the referring physician, in Manual of Psychiatric Consultation and Emergency Care. Edited by Guggenheim FG, Weiner MF. New York, Jason Aronson, 1984, pp 115–123

Renner JA Jr: Drug addiction, in Massachusetts General Hospital Handbook of General Hospital Psychiatry, 2nd Edition. Edited by Hackett TP, Cassem NH. Littleton, MA, PSG Publishers, 1987, pp 29–41

Slaby AE, Cullen LO: Dementia and delirium, in Principles of Medical Psychiatry. Edited by Stoudemire MD, Fogel BS. Orlando, FL, Grune & Stratton, 1987, pp 135–175

Stone AA: The Tarasoff case and some of its progeny: suing psychotherapists to safeguard society, in Law, Psychiatry, and Morality. Washington, DC, American Psychiatric Press, 1984, pp 161–190

Strain JJ: The intrafamilial environment of the chronically ill patient, in Psychological Interventions in Medical Practice. Edited by Strain JJ. New York, Appleton-Century-Crofts, 1978, pp 151–171

Strain JJ, Grossman S: Psychological reactions to medical illness and hospitalization, in Psychological Care of the Medically Ill. Edited by Strain JJ, Grossman S. New York, Appleton-Century-Crofts, 1975, pp 23–36

Yager J: Cognitive aspects of illness, in Consultation-Liaison Psychiatry. Edited by Pasnau RO. New York, Grune & Stratton, 1975, pp 61–71

8

Writing Up the Consultation

A written psychiatric consultation on a general-hospital inpatient unit is a unique medical document. Like the usual medical record, it contains the history, examination, and the physician's impression of the patient (Dean 1963). But unlike the medical record, it is not written only to supplement the physician's memory or to provide a legal record. The written consultation includes a therapeutic plan, yet does not constitute official orders for nursing or house staff to carry out. It involves not just the patient's concerns, but also—and especially—the questions asked by the primary physician about the patient's diagnosis and care. It is an official doctor-to-doctor communication.

The content and form of the written psychiatric consultation must serve the function of answering the expressed questions of the primary physician, whether or not the physician, the patient, or the staff is the primary focus of the consult. As such, the document is formally addressed to the patient's primary physician. However, it must be written discreetly, with the knowledge that it is available to the patient by law. Additionally, the consultation must be written with a broad audience in mind, because it is designed to be used by the entire treatment team, which variously may include nurses, social workers, and specialty therapists and their students. Finally, it is unavoidably available to others—appropriately and inappropriately—such as insurance companies and hospital review committees.

This chapter is organized into sections corresponding to the suggested sections for a written psychiatric consultation and other medical documents (see Appendix A):

- Title
- Date, time, and sources of information
- Identifying statement
- History
- Mental status examination
- Formulations
- Recommendations

Note, however, that this format is considerably different from other reports such as legal consultations (Hoffman 1986) and disability evaluations (Okpaku 1988). The written consultation may be supplemented by a computer-assisted data base (Appendix B) that facilitates patient tracking, research, and quality assurance (Hammer et al. 1984, 1985). We do not discuss a wide variety of consultation styles. Instead, we offer a scheme, as well as the rationale underlying each suggestion. Certain issues come up again and again in the consideration of the written psychiatric consultation, including the consultation audience, confidentiality, the indivisibility of mind and body, psychiatry as a bona fide and useful specialty, the use of technical language, and the importance of the consultant-consultee and doctor-patient collaborative relationships. Mindful of these issues, we offer the following scheme, which contains the elements the consultant can use to facilitate his or her effective communication in the written consultation document. We attempt to capture a balance between an extensively detailed format and a skeletal outline.

WRITTEN PSYCHIATRIC CONSULTATION DOCUMENT

Title

The written consultation should be given a title, even when a printed general consultation form is used. The consultation is addressed to a staff bombarded by many sources of information, all vying for their attention. The title facilitates the location of specific desired and/or needed information among the usual welter of progress and nursing notes, laboratory reports, and other consultation documents. The title should include some form of the word "psychiatry," your rank or position (resident, attending, intern), and the appropriate descriptive term ("consultation," "note," "preliminary note," "workup," and/or "follow-up").

Often there are several stages of written communication. You may receive the consultation request, discuss it with the referring physician, review the chart, and then find that the patient is away from the ward or is sedated or otherwise indisposed. A titled preliminary note informs the service that you are involved, interested, and available, and has some preliminary data about the case. Similarly titled written notes are an integral part of the consultant's follow-up visits (contracts made) with the patient, the family, and the service.

Date, Time, and Sources of Information

Next to the title of each note are the date and the time the note was written and a list of the sources of information used by the consultant. This serves three purposes: (1) it conforms to the medical style; (2) it informs the consultee of the old and new chart review and of interviews performed by the consultant; and (3) it records the data base for the consultant's conclusions and identifies resource persons, family, and other medical staff. Recording the length and number of visits underscores the time and effort expended, even when the written note is short. (This may also be relevant to quality assurance, billing, and insurance transactions.)

Identifying Statement

The opening sentences of the note set the tone of the consultation. The psychiatrist must (1) distill all of the data about the patient into a succinctly worded summary of the patient's presenting condition, and (2) clarify the often vague explicit and implicit demands of the referring service, thereby formulating a question that includes a consideration of each of these elements.

After assimilating all of the explicit and implicit information related to the clinical problem, begin your remarks with a focus on those facts about the patient that are most relevant to the immediate problem. These facts, like those entered at the beginning of a written history, are worded in the familiar medical style, but they are selected with a view to the formulations and recommendations to follow: "We are asked to see this socially isolated, needy 60-year-old woman with a history of unexplained multiple admissions for diabetic ketoacidosis—this 32-year-old man with a bleeding ulcer, whose mother recently died—this 45-year-old man with headaches, whose delinquent son was recently incarcerated—this 26-year-old woman, admitted for a hysterectomy because of pelvic adhesions and pain, who has a long history of surgical procedures in several institutions for various diagnoses, without relief of symptoms."

The next sentence or clause restates in a workable fashion the observations and diagnostic, therapeutic, and/or management problems that occasioned the request for a consultation. The wording of this request as received by the consultant is not uncommonly as vague as "R/O [rule out] schizophrenia." This reflects the psychologically unsophisticated and/or resistant (Krakowski 1971, 1974) state of the primary physician's thinking about the psychophysiological functioning of the patient, and often engenders annoyance and sarcasm on the part of the consultant. There is no place, however, in the opening or any other part of the written consultation for expressing any feelings other than those due a professional colleague who has paid the consultant the respect of making a referral. It is useful to begin with a statement to the effect that a psychiatric evaluation has been requested and then to detail what seem to the psychiatrist to be the events or behaviors that precipitated the referral. Whether or not these observations—not interpretations—are offered explicitly in the referral, they are the formulation of the psychiatrist's approach to the consultee-consultant contract. An example of such a statement is, "Psychiatric evaluation is now requested because of a change in the patient's mood, alertness, and cognition occurring over the last week," or, "The patient's daily crying spells since admission are of concern to the service."

At this point, the question of whether to use psychiatric technical language may arise (Engel et al. 1957; Kaufman 1953; Krakowski 1973). (The consultant's facility with biomedical language is generally not problematic and may be beneficial.) A broad range of styles may be useful, depending on the circumstances—for example, the psychiatric sophistication of the consultee, the need for descriptive accuracy, the tendency to view psychiatric labels as pejorative, the potential for education, and clinical emergencies. Psychiatry, like other medical disciplines, has evolved a specialized terminology that reflects continuing efforts at descriptive and theoretical precision. The consultant's task is to strike a balance between oversimplification and technical obfuscation. In general, as in all writing, the aim is to be as clear, direct, and concise as possible. Technical terms should be used when necessary. A nonjudgmental definition of the term can be unobtrusively inserted. The consultee is seeking an expert opinion as well as one that he or she can understand and apply.

It is important to consider for whom (Krakowski 1971) the consultation is being written. The consultation formally exists as a doctor-to-doctor communication. It is seldom a personal letter, especially when written in a hospital record. The request for consultation itself may have been instigated by someone other than the attending physician—by someone less involved in the care of the patient, such as a nurse, another consultant, or a relative, who awaits the impressions of the psychiatric expert (Kimball 1973). The issue of responsibility and confidentiality in the consultation process has been thoughtfully considered by Kimball (1979) and others (Engelhardt and McCullough 1979). In any event, the written consultation is meant to be read, for clinical and educational purposes, by many people and is available, for currently unavoidable reasons, to many others, who may read it for insurance or review purposes, for legal purposes, out of idle curiosity, or even out of maliciousness.

The ultimate clause or sentence is the consultant's formulation of the problem to which the rest of the document will be addressed. The consultant might note (to pursue some of the examples we have used), "For the purpose of differentiating an organic brain syndrome from a depression" or "Psychiatric evaluation is now requested to delineate the etiology and pathogenesis of this possible depression, and the treatment options and recommendation." The consultee's appreciation for the clear reformulation of the patient's problem generally outweighs any passing annoyance at his or her statements being paraphrased. The overriding necessity is to ask a question that is answerable, if only by a carefully explained "I don't know." As we have already mentioned, the consultee's optimism and anxiety may be all-embracing and overwhelming. Dealing with these feelings tactfully and focusing requests are central goals both of ongoing psychiatric liaison and of communications concerning individual consultation. The restatement and formulation of the consultee's request, once accepted, acknowledges the contract between consultee and consultant.

History

The psychiatric consultant's written history of the patient's present illness is a chronologically organized presentation of the interrelated life events—medical, social, and interpersonal—that bear directly on the current problem. The technique of psychiatric history taking and writing has been considered in depth in the literature relevant to the training of psychiatrists. Several considerations deserve specific attention in the writing of a consultation.

The first consideration is the issue of confidentiality (discussed earlier in this chapter). In writing the history, decide which of the sensitive communications of the patient or others are essential pieces of information for the treatment team so that they may pursue a more successful interaction with the patient. The issue is a complex one and is best handled in active collaboration with the informant in terms of what you will and will not communicate to the consultee and/or others. This discussion may not absolve you from fulfilling your clinical responsibilities to the consultee, which may include divulging previous medical history about abortions, antisocial behaviors, and psychiatric illness. VIP patients and those personally, as well as professionally, known to primary or consulting physicians present delicate problems. The overriding consideration will be the welfare of the patient.

Another issue is that of weighing completeness against immediate clinical relevance. Physicians are trained to be highly invested in thorough documentation. While this tradition is reasonable and often important, the consultee frequently perceives extensive consultations as peripheral to the patient's care. A long, detailed report may simply leave the focus of the psychiatric evaluation to the chance scanning of the consultee. In those circumstances where a more thorough workup is considered useful, a typed report assures a greater chance of being read than does a handwritten one.

Another special quality of the psychiatric consultation history is that it aims both to teach other medical professionals about psychosomatic aspects of illness in general and to foster understanding of a particular patient (Kimball 1979). A formal psychiatric review of systems can serve these simultaneous ends. This review includes medical conditions; ongoing pharmacotherapy and other forms of therapy; recent stresses and anniversaries of previous losses; the state of social, family, and work satisfaction; and characteristic patterns of response to stress and their relationship to past medical or psychiatric illnesses. It is frequently important to cite negative as well as positive findings. Viewing the patient's present behaviors in the context of his or her psychosocial history, stressful life events, characteristic defenses, and behavior styles helps the primary physician translate frustration into purposeful therapeutic activity (Goldiamond and Dyrud 1968). This understanding improves the doctor-patient relationship and may provide such a solid underpinning for the psychiatrist's formulations and recommendations that their presentation seems almost superfluous. The following vignette illustrates this point:

> A 32-year-old woman was hospitalized for treatment of several vaguely described complaints of pain. She expressed massive hostility and anxiety to the whole staff and invoked in them a similar reaction. She had a highly developed ability to play on people's vulnerabilities and insecurities. She accused the staff of abandonment and malpractice and asserted that she was considering filing a lawsuit. The staff's enraged, helpless, and avoidant responses only fed into this vicious cycle. The consultant's history was an explication of the patient's lifetime of isolation, depression, and poor communication. Without further direction from the psychiatrist, the staff's annoyance turned to pity, their stance softened, and the working relationship improved so dramatically that an overlooked pneumonia and pleuritis were diagnosed and successfully treated.

Mental Status Examination

The mental status examination tends to be ignored. Its skillful documentation by a psychiatric consultant underscores its *necessity* as a component of a medical workup (Langsley 1979). The examination educates the consultees in its performance and provides a baseline for future diagnosis and care of the patient, as well as the vital data base for correct management. It demonstrates that psychiatrists, like other medical specialists, base their conclusions on an orderly series of evaluations. Moreover, serial mental status examinations can often chart important signs along the course of an illness. Although other schemes are available, we find it useful to include the following aspects of the patient: appearance, verbal behavior, affect, thought flow and content, sensorium/cognition, intellectual capacity and function, insight, and judgment. Listing these categories serves to remind the consultant and educate the consultee about how to organize their thinking about a patient's mental status. The use and straightforward explanation of technical terms in this context also furthers these functions. Normal findings at the time of one examination may prove to be either an improvement on, or a deterioration of, the patient's usual functioning. In any case, they provide a vital baseline against which any changes in these findings can be identified.

In this context, it may be necessary to spell out the examinations that were performed and the details of the results. For example, in an 82-year-old patient with "altered mental status," we noted, "Oriented to person, place, and time; unable to remember three objects at 5 minutes; could spell 'cat' and 'hand' forward but not 'hand' backward; and a face-hand test was positive, indicating diffuse cortical dysfunction." Many of the important elements of clinically valid mental status examinations have been discussed by Strub and Black (1981) and by Folstein and colleagues (1975). The examination's clinical validity is complicated by its exquisite sensitivity to the interviewer's tone and style and the patient's attitudes, expectations, and fears about both psychiatry and his or her cognitive functioning. The evaluation also identifies the patient's physical and emotional comfort, ability to attend to and cooperate with an interviewer called in by someone else, and the overall and immediate circumstances (including physiologic energy level and drug effects) of the patient. For example, a regressed, backward, severely disabled patient showed a dramatic improvement in mental status after being bathed, shaved, nicely dressed, and taken away from the ward for examination. Thus, it is important for the consultant both to record the state of the patient at the time of the interview and to explicitly educate the consultee about its clinical influence.

When therapy, including pharmacotherapy, is to be instituted, a carefully documented mental status examination will inform physicians who see the patient in the future of the indications that led to the therapeutic decision. A patient successfully in treatment for a major psychiatric illness may appear to be so normal that the successful and necessary therapy might be prematurely and abruptly withdrawn.

This view of the mental status examination as a useful tool rather than a required exercise, and as a system for assessing the patient's functioning at a particular moment in time (similar to any other medical examination) rather than a fixed quality, makes for more reasoned, explicit, and accurate diagnostic formulations in general. For example, a consultant summoned by a gastroenterologist reviewed the chart of a 38-year-old woman admitted for treatment of irritable bowel syndrome. Review of the old chart revealed eight psychiatric consultations in the past 8 years, each with a different diagnosis. These labels ranged from "hysterical character" and "obsessional character" to "schizophrenia." After careful review of the past mental status examinations to determine the criteria for each diagnosis, the consultant was able to explain to the treating service staff that the patient could most usefully be understood as having a borderline character disorder and as manifesting widely varying symptoms at various points in her unstable existence.

Formulations

The formulations pose the most delicate problems in writing the consultation. The choice of the term "formulations" rather than the more traditional medical "diagnosis" or even "differential diagnosis" highlights the issue. Offering a neat diagnostic label may provide a tidy ending not only to the document but also to careful consideration of the patient and to the human interaction of patient and medical-care team. The situation is similar to that in other medical specialties, when a human being with a constellation of complaints and findings becomes a "diabetic" or a "missed abortion." Psychiatric labels are poorly understood and anxiety-provoking, and frequently put distance between consultant, consultee, and patient. However, diagnostic labels follow a medical tradition, help in structuring a set of observations or a differential diagnosis, and are sometimes required by insurance companies and regulatory agencies. In some insurance payment schemes currently in vogue, such diagnoses may allow reimbursement to the hospital at a much higher rate than without the diagnosis. In these cases, the consultant can use a DSM-III-R formulation and number and explain it in the written consultation. (This is an opportunity to acquaint the consultee with DSM-III-R as a reference and as a demonstration of psychiatry's move toward greater diagnostic precision.)

Sometimes a final diagnosis cannot be made at the time of consultation because certain data are lacking. This situation needs to be specifically identified to the consultee. For example, additional criteria for schizophrenic and affective disorders may require further observation of the illness over a specified time span. The psychiatrist is frequently consulted to decide whether the patient's pain is organic or functional and can only conclude (Lazerson 1976) after careful examination that it is neither—or both. The patient may have started out with an injury, but weeks or months of pain, spasm, anxiety, accommodations in life-style, and reactions in friends, relatives, and lawyers, obscure the clinical picture by the time the patient is admitted for a workup.

A discussion of the dynamics of the patient as an individual in the medical-care situation is the most clinically useful summary of the consultant's findings. In the case of the patient with borderline character disorder described earlier, the psychiatrist wrote the following:

> The patient desperately wants encouragement and support from others, but is unable to express her needs directly and successfully. At times the patient is driven to make human contact by dramatic complaints and seductive behavior; at other times she withdraws into rigidly controlled and controlling ritualistic behavior. When she fails and feels disliked, she may become so upset that she falls apart completely and is unable to function.

Given this shift in understanding, the primary service staff's behavior changed from avoidance to approach, and the patient's behavior, while erratic, no longer was such an obstacle to her care.

Recommendations

The recommendations (or suggestions or treatment) section is sometimes the only and often the first one that the consultee actually reads. In this section he or she hopes to find the answer to the problem, the fulfillment or embodiment of the implicit and explicit contracts between consultant and consultee. Like the contract, its tone is confident, informative, and respectful of the professionalism of the recipient. Its content is scientific, reasonable, and practical. The recommendations constitute a comprehensive approach to the clinical problem and a careful delineation of immediate and long-term management. For completeness, you may also indicate important components of the approach that have already been performed, or which of those remaining to be performed you are assuming responsibility for and when and how the consultee will be apprised of results.

The following is a suggested conceptual scheme for organizing the recommendations (see next chapter for further detail).

Further Workup. Further workup may be required to clarify the diagnosis, precipitating events, and/or resources. It may include laboratory tests for the diagnosis of abnormalities, whether these tests are primary, such as serum alcohol level, or contributory, such as hematocrit. Workup also may require more history or history from other sources, such as old medical records, school files, employers, friends, and relatives. For example, a diagnosis of sleep apnea is often strongly suspected on the basis of the bed partner's report of loud snoring, apneic periods, and gross physical restlessness. The psychiatric consultant may also point out the need for consultation by other specialists.

Consultee Management. The second category of recommendations is management by the consultee. These recommendations may include pharmacologic, social, psychotherapeutic, situational, and/or legal management. The consultant may suggest the manipulation of drugs that are administered for the patient's primary conditions but produce side effects, such as impotence and drowsiness, that are relevant to the consultation problem. He or she may recommend administration or withdrawal of psychotropic medication. Specific detailed regimens should be suggested in the latter case, along with therapeutic and side effects to be anticipated. This is an effective way to communicate the medical relevance of psychiatry.

Examples of legal management recommendations include ways of explaining a procedure to a patient to obtain and document informed consent and ways of determining legal mental competence. It is important to help the consultee differentiate medical/ psychiatric questions from medicolegal ones. This may involve calling and quoting the hospital's lawyer or suggesting that the consultee do so. Management of social workers, visiting nurses, public-aid workers, and the chaplain or for assisting the patient in obtaining special equipment, such as wheelchairs, home dialysis equipment, or other special care devices, is often pivotal in ensuring successful aftercare. Such suggestions serve to guide the primary physician's attention toward holistic care (Strain 1978) rather than just symptom relief.

The lines between situational, psychological, and psychotherapeutic interventions are sometimes difficult to draw (Engel 1980). There is a conceptual continuum. At one end is structuring, ordering the environment and schedule of the disoriented patient with an organic brain syndrome, arranging for an interpreter for a frightened non-English-speaking patient, or obtaining permission for supporting relatives to remain with and care for the patient.

In the middle of the continuum are recommendations for dealing with problems occasioned by the patient's character structure and response to the medical setting. A classic example is limit setting. An outline of the rationale and regimen for dealing with an abusive, constantly demanding, or engaging but draining patient and its implementation have a dramatically soothing effect on the service staff. The consultant thus channels frustrated feelings provoked by the patient into constructive behavior by the patient and staff, such as setting up a schedule of frequent but structured patient contacts or instructions about how, when, and why to call in hospital guards or the police (Groves 1975).

Next along the spectrum are recommendations for a general approach to the patient based on an understanding of character structure. For those patients who are acutely sensitive to power issues, you may suggest that the primary physician explain and phrase all orders in terms of choices. With other patients, who are overwhelmed by ambivalence, the caregivers may make a contract to offer straightforward recommendations. You may stress the need to reinforce the patient's desirable behaviors, downplaying preoccupations with symptoms and helplessness and underscoring attempts to assume responsibility. You can use personal knowledge of the primary physician's personality style by taking this, too, into account in framing this kind of recommendation.

The other end of the spectrum is the recommendation for formal psychotherapy. You may recommend that the consultee encourage the patient to follow through on suggested psychotherapy or suggest that a member of the primary medical team begin or continue a limited psychotherapeutic process. An experienced and sophisticated nonpsychiatric medical professional may wish and be able to do limited psychotherapy. Others on the medical team may use psychotherapeutic techniques for a patient who needs support and ventilation. These interventions may be on a one-to-one basis or may involve the patient's family. You may offer advice as to the frequency, length, and duration of these sessions.

Consultant Management. The third main category of recommendations is management by the consultant or care by a specialist in psychiatry. This category is largely self-explanatory. It includes recommendations for inpatient psychiatric hospitalization, outpatient psychotherapies, and behavioral, psychodynamic, hypnotic, and/or somatic psychiatric therapy (e.g., ECT, pharmacotherapy, biofeedback). If a referral to another psychiatrist is advised, the precise mechanism must be specified. When the consultant will continue to evaluate the patient, this needs to be agreed upon and specified. If no psychiatric follow-up is indicated at the time, this may be stated, along with an invitation to contact the consultant or a suitable substitute when necessary.

The consultation then ends with an expression of your appreciation for the referral and your legible or retyped signature and phone number. Making your availability manifest is tangible evidence of the physician's professional responsibility.

THE LIMITED, NONCOMPREHENSIVE CONSULTATION

Situations arise in which the usual complete psychiatric evaluation is not requested and/or indicated. These consultations are termed "limited." The medical or psychiatric picture may be emergent. The situation in which the time available for workup is limited by the patient's condition, treatments, or imminent discharge is often a loaded situation and worthy of fuller discussion elsewhere. It may be immediately clear that the patient needs inpatient psychiatric care. The treating service may have a specific limited request for advice or information, for example, "Will treatment with steroids pose a danger to this patient, who has a history of a schizophrenic break in the distant past?" In these cases, you have a right and duty first to decide as an independent physician whether a limited consultation is appropriate and then to clearly and accurately title the written document for medical and legal clarity. Otherwise, the conceptual framework for deciding content, tone, and style is the same as that for a comprehensive consultation.

LEGAL IMPLICATIONS

In the current litigious era, the psychiatric consultation document serves important purposes of providing data for future quality assurance and legal reviews. Information about suicidality, homicidality, baseline mental status, and competence is essential. These issues (to be adressed in greater detail in Chapter 12) may also have important bearing on medical procedures such as resuscitation, consent or refusal to give consent, and discharge to independent living.

CONCLUSIONS

We have tried in this detailed dissection of the anatomy of the psychiatric consultation document to share our growing awareness of the profundity and complexity of the issues involved in writing a consultation. These issues are often extensions of those faced by a liaison psychiatrist verbally managing a consultation. Although the array of delicate and demanding questions may seem formidable, our aim is not to overwhelm, but rather to impress the reader with the range of choices and possibilities for having a constructive impact in the written record as distinct from other liaison interactions. A psychiatric consultation is a rare opportunity not only to help a patient and doctor in distress but also to communicate effective, lasting, implicit, and explicit messages about psychiatric theory and practice and about psychiatrists as experts, colleagues, and individuals.

REFERENCES

Dean ES: Writing psychiatric reports. Am J Psychiatry 119:759–762, 1963

Engel GL: The clinical application of the biopsychosocial model. Am J Psychiatry 137:535–544, 1980

Engel GL, Green WL Jr, Reichsman F, et al: A graduate and undergraduate teaching program on the psychological aspects of medicine. J Med Educ 32:859–870, 1957

Engelhardt HT Jr, McCullough LB: Confidentiality in the consultation-liaison process: ethical dimensions and conflicts. Psychiatr Clin North Am 2:403–413, 1979

Folstein MF, Folstein SE, McHugh PR: Mini-Mental State: a practical method for grading the cognitive state of patients for the clinician. J Psychiatr Res 12:189–198, 1975

Goldiamond I, Dyrud J: Some applications and implications of behavioral analysis for psychotherapy, in Research in Psychotherapy, Vol 3. Edited by Schlien J. Washington, DC, American Psychological Association, 1968, pp 54–89

Groves J: Management of the borderline patient on a medical or surgical ward: the psychiatric consultant's role. Int J Psychiatry Med 6:337–348, 1975

Hammer JS, Lyons JS, Strain JJ: Micro-Cares: an information management system for psychosocial services in hospital settings. Proceedings SCAMC, Vol 8, 1984, pp 234–237

Hammer J, Hammond D, Strain J, et al: Microcomputers and consultation psychiatry in the general hospital. Gen Hosp Psychiatry 7:119–124, 1985

Hoffman BF: How to write a psychiatric report for litigation following a personal injury. Am J Psychiatry 143:164–169, 1986

Kaufman MR: The role of the psychiatrist in the general hospital. Psychiatr Q 27:367–381, 1953

Kimball CP: Liaison psychiatry in the university medical center. Compr Psychiatry 14:241–249, 1973

Kimball CP: The issue of confidentiality in the consultation-liaison process, in The Teaching of Psychosomatic Medicine and Consultation-Liaison Psychiatry. Edited by Kimball CP, Krakowski AJ. Bibliotheca Psychiatrica No. 159. Basel, S Karger, 1979, pp 82–89

Krakowski AJ: Doctor-doctor relationship. Psychosomatics 12:11–15, 1971

Krakowski AJ: Doctor-doctor relationship. III. A study of feelings influencing the vocation and its tasks. Psychosomatics 14:156–161, 1973

Krakowski AJ: Consultation psychiatry, present global status: a survey. Psychother Psychosom 23:78–86, 1974

Langsley DG: The mental status examination, in Psychiatry in General Medical Practice. Edited by Usdin G, Lewis JM. New York, McGraw-Hill, 1979, pp 22–38

Lazerson AM: The psychiatrist in primary medical care training: a solution to the mind-body dichotomy? Am J Psychiatry 133:964–966, 1976

Okpaku SO: The psychiatrist and the social security disability insurance and supplemental security income programs. Hosp Community Psychiatry 39:879–883, 1988

Strain JJ: Psychological Interventions in Medical Practice. New York, Appleton-Century-Crofts, 1978

Strub RL, Black FW: Organic Brain Syndromes: An Introduction to Neurobehavioral Disorders. Philadelphia, PA, FA Davis, 1981, pp 39–86

APPENDIX A: SUGGESTED OUTLINE FOR THE WRITTEN PSYCHIATRIC CONSULTATION

1. Title: specialty, rank, full or limited note

2. Date, time, and sources of information

3. Identifying statement:
   a. Psychosocial information having bearing on the patient's overall condition (e.g., chronic schizophrenia, mental retardation, recent bereavement or divorce)
   b. Distillation of the contract between consultee and consultant
   c. Chief concern of consultee

4. History
   a. History of the present psychiatric illness
   b. Medical history, with pertinent data
      i. Chart review
      ii. Relationship between medical and psychiatric findings
      iii. Educating the medical staff on issues to consider in this patient and in other patients with psychiatric signs and symptoms

5. Mental status examination

6. Formulations

7. Recommendations

8. Special circumstances
   a. Legal consultations
   b. Time- or issue-limited consultations

Appendix B: An Example of a Computer-Assisted Data Base As A Supplement To The Written Consultation[1]

MICRO-CARES™ CONSORTIUM PSYCHIATRIC CONSULTATION QUESTIONNAIRE

USE NO. 2 PENCIL ONLY

Proper Mark ●   Improper Marks ⊗ ⊘ ◐

INSTRUCTIONS: Please mark the most appropriate choice for each question, except where multiple answers are specifically requested. Print the numbers in the write-in spaces above the corresponding responses.

SITE CODE   PRACT. CODE

PATIENT NAME (PLEASE PRINT)

DATE OF ADMISSION — MO DAY YEAR

DATE OF CONSULT REQUEST — MO DAY YEAR

ADMITTED FROM
1. Home
2. Med. Hosp. or Nursing Home
3. Psych. Hosp. or Institution
4. Undomiciled
5. Other
6. Unknown

PATIENT TYPE
1. Inpatient
2. Outpatient

BILLING CODE
1. Medicare
2. Commercial/BlueCross
3. Self Pay
4. Workman's Compensation
5. Public Aid/Agency
6. Does not apply
7. Other
8. Unknown

TIME OF CONSULT REQUEST

DATE OF FIRST VISIT — MO DAY YEAR

TIME OF FIRST VISIT

TIME SPENT ON FIRST VISIT
1. None
2. 1-14 mins
3. 15-30 mins
4. 31-60 mins
5. > 60 mins

URGENCY
1. Immediate
2. Today
3. Routine
4. Unknown

SEX — Male / Female

REFERRING SERVICE (See Codes P.2)

PATIENT NUMBER

AGE

CURRENT MARITAL STATUS
1. Single/Never Married
2. (Re)Married
3. Separated
4. Divorced
5. Widowed
6. Unknown

RACE/ETHNICITY
1. White
2. Black
3. Oriental
4. Hispanic
5. Other
6. Unknown

RELIGION
1. Protestant
2. Catholic
3. Jewish
4. Other
5. None
6. Unknown

EMPLOYMENT STATUS
1. Full-time
2. Part-time
3. Unemployed
4. Unemp'd (Disabled)
5. Retired
6. Other
7. Unknown
8. Does not apply

EDUCATION (highest level completed)
1. Grad-Prof degree
2. College grad
3. Partial college
4. HS/GED/vo-tech
5. Partial Hi.School
6. Junior High School
7. Less than 7 years
8. Unknown
9. Does not apply

USUAL OCCUPATION CLASS
1. High executive, large proprietor, major professional
2. Business manager, medium proprietor, lesser professional
3. Administrative personnel, small proprietor, minor professional
4. Clerical & Sales worker, little proprietor, technician
5. Skilled manual employee
6. Machine operator, semi-skilled employee
7. Unskilled or homemaker
8. Student
9. None
10. Unknown

PLEASE DO NOT MARK IN THIS AREA   090105

---

[1] Reprinted with permission of the Magnum Medical Software Corporation, Chicago, Illinois.

CODE TRANSLATIONS

REFERRING SERVICE										
Anesthesia	= 01	General Surg.	= 19	Neurology	= 08	Orthopedics	= 12	Preventive Med	= 02
Card/Thor Surg	= 22	Gynecology	= 09	Neurosurgery	= 10	Otolaryngol.	= 13	Psychiatry	= 17
Dentistry	= 04	Hospice	= 27	Obstetrics	= 20	Pathology	= 14	Radiology	= 18
Dermatology	= 03	Infect. Dis.	= 06	Oncology	= 26	Pediatrics	= 15	Renal Medicine	= 07
Emergency Room	= 21	Medicine	= 05	Opthalmol.	= 11	Physical Med	= 16	Urology	= 24
	= 28		= 29					Plastic Surg.	= 23	OTHER	= 25

KARNOFSKY SCALE: ESTIMATE FUNCTIONING DURING THE ONE MONTH PRIOR TO ADMISSION AND AT TERMINATION EXAM.

ABLE TO CARRY ON NORMALLY. NO SPECIAL CARE IS NECESSARY	99%	Normal, no complaints, no evidence of disease.
	90%	Normal activity. Minor signs/symptoms of disease.
	80%	Normal activity with effort. Some signs/symptoms of disease.
UNABLE TO WORK BUT ABLE TO LIVE AT HOME & CARE FOR MOST PERSONAL NEEDS	70%	Cares for self, but can't perform normal activity or work.
	60%	Cares for self, but needs occasional assistance.
	50%	Requires considerable assistance and frequent medical care.
UNABLE TO CARE FOR SELF. NEEDS INSTITUTIONAL OR HOSPITAL CARE. DISEASE IS RAPIDLY PROGRESSING.	40%	Moderately disabled; requires special care/assistance.
	30%	Sever.disabled; possible hospitalization; death not imminent.
	20%	Very sick. Hospitalization necessary.
	10%	Moribund with a fatal process progressing rapidly.
	0%	Died or will die within the week.

PSYCHOTROPIC MEDICATION RECOMMENDED, STATUS, AND ADVERSE REACTIONS

New = Agent started after patient arrived in hospital.

Old = Agent patient was taking at time of entry to hospital.

STATUS
1 New/Recc and Taken
2 New/Recc and Not Taken
3 New/Recc/Taken-Discontinued
4 New/Recc/Unknown
5 Old/Taken
6 Old/Discontinued
7 Old/Unknown

REACTIONS
1 Somatic/Definite
2 Somatic/Suspected
3 Psych./Definite
4 Psych./Suspected
5 No Adverse Reaction
6 Unknown
7 Does not apply

CODES	ANTIANXIETY MEDICATION	
101	Alprazolam	XANAX
102	Chlordiazepoxide hydrochloride	LIBRIUM
102	Chlordiazepoxide hydrochloride	LIBRITABS
103	Clorazepate dipotassium	TRANXENE-SD
103	Clorazepate dipotassium	TRANXENE
104	Diazepam	VALIUM
104	Diazepam	VALRELEASE
105	Halazepam	PAXIPAM
106	Hydroxyzine hydrochloride	ATARAX
106	Hydroxyzine hydrochloride	ATARAX 100
106	Hydroxyzine hydrochloride	VISTARIL INTRAMUSC.
107	Hydroxyzine pamoate	VISTARIL
108	Lorazepam	ATIVAN
109	Meprobamate	EQUANIL
110	Oxazepam	SERAX
111	Prazepam	CENTRAX
112	OTHER	

CODES	ANTIDEPRESSANT MEDICATION	
201	Amitriptyline hydrochloride	ELAVIL
201	Amitriptyline hydrochloride	ENDEP
202	Amoxapine	ASENDIN
203	Chlordiazep. & amitript.hydroch.	LIMBITROL
204	Desipramine hydrochloride	NORPRAMIN
205	Doxepin hydrochloride	SINEQUAN
205	Doxepin hydrochloride	ADAPIN
206	Imipramine hydrochloride	TOFRANIL
207	Imipramine pamoate	TOFRANIL-PM
208	Isocarboxazid	MARPLAN
209	Maprotiline hydrochloride	LUDIOMIL
210	Nortriptyline hydrochloride	PAMELOR
211	Perphenaz. & amitript.hydroch.	TRIAVIL
211	Perphenaz. & amitript.hydroch.	ETRAFON
212	Phenelzine sulfate	NARDIL
213	Protryptyline hydrochloride	VIVACTIL
214	Tranylcypramine sulfate	PARNATE
215	Trazodone hydrochloride	DESYREL
216	Trimipramine maleate	SURMONTIL
217	Fluoxetine hydrochloride	PROZAC
218	OTHER	

CODES	ANTIMANIC MEDICATION	
301	Lithium carbonate	ESKALITH
301	Lithium carbonate	ESKALITH-CR
301	Lithium carbonate	LITHOBID
302	Lithium citrate	CIBALITH-S
303	OTHER	

	ANTIPSYCHOTIC MEDICATION	
401	Chlorpromazine hydrochloride	THORAZINE
402	Fluphenazine hydrochloride	PERMITIL
402	Fluphenazine hydrochloride	PROLIXIN
403	Haloperidol	HALDOL
404	Loxapine hydrochloride	LOXITANE IM
404	Loxapine hydrochloride	LOXITANE C
405	Loxapine succinate	LOXITANE
406	Perphenazine	TRILAFON
407	Prochlorperazine	COMPAZINE
408	Thioridazine	MELLARIL-S
409	Thioridazine hydrochloride	MELLARIL
410	Thiothixene	NAVANE
411	Trifluoperazine hydrochloride	STELAZINE
412	OTHER	

	SEDATIVES, HYPNOTICS, ANTICONVULSANTS	
501	Phenobarbital	PHENOBARBITAL
502	Phenobarbital sodium	PHENO. SODIUM
503	Ethchlorvynol	PLACIDYL
504	Flurazepam hydrochloride	DALMANE
505	Mephobarbital	MEBARAL
506	Methyprylon	NOLUDAR 300
506	Methyprylon	NOLUDAR
507	Pentobarbital	NEMBUTAL EXLIXIR
508	Pentobarbital sodium	NEMB.SODIUM CAPS
508	Pentobarbital sodium	NEMB.SOD.SUPPOS.
509	Secobarbital sodium	SECONAL SODIUM
510	Temazepam	RESTORIL
511	Triazolam	HALCION
512	Diphenylhydantoin	DILANTIN
513	Carbamazipine	TEGRETOL
514	OTHER	

PRIMARY	LIVING
INCOME	**WITH**
SOURCE	① Self only
① Earned (self/spouse)	② Parent(s) only
② Social Security/Retirement	③ Parent(s) & minor
③ Social Security/Disability	④ Spouse only
④ Supplemental Security Income	⑤ Spouse & minor
⑤ Public Aid	⑥ Other Adult only
⑥ Unemployment compensation benefits	⑦ Other Adult & minor
⑦ Family	⑧ Nursing home or institution
⑧ Savings/Investments	⑨ Minor(s) only
⑨ Workmen's Compensation	
⑩ Other	⑩ Other
⑪ None	⑪ Unknown
⑫ Unknown	

PSYCHIATRIC DIAGNOSIS AXIS I AND II
IR = Init/Rule Out   TR = Term/Rule Out
IC = Init/Confirmed   TC = Term/Confirmed

LIFE EVENTS IN LAST YEAR: Answer Y = Yes, N = No, U = Unknown

1. Serious Med. illness (SELF) .... Ⓨ Ⓝ Ⓤ
2. Serious Med. illness (SIG. OTHER) .... Ⓨ Ⓝ Ⓤ
3. Major Psych. treatment (SELF) .... Ⓨ Ⓝ Ⓤ
4. Major Psych. treatment (SIG. OTHER) . Ⓨ Ⓝ Ⓤ
5. Death of significant other ..... Ⓨ Ⓝ Ⓤ
6. Divorce or separation .... Ⓨ Ⓝ Ⓤ
7. Job loss (SELF OR SIG. OTHER) Ⓨ Ⓝ Ⓤ
8. OTHER .... Ⓨ Ⓝ Ⓤ

REASONS/PROBLEMS FOR
THE CONSULT STATED BY: CONSULTANT ─┐
(Check up to 5 per column)   CONSULTEE ─┘

1. Alcohol problems .... ① ②
2. Antisocial acts (lying/crimes).............................. ① ②
3. Anxiety/fear .... ① ②
4. Behavioral management/agitation .... ① ②
5. Behavior (strange/unexplained/bizarre) .... ① ②
6. Bowel problems .... ① ②
7. Child abuse .... ① ②
8. Coping problems .... ① ②
9. Depression .... ① ②
10. Diagnosis (suspected psychological component) .... ① ②
11. Drug problems .... ① ②
12. Eating disorder .... ① ②
13. Ethical issues .... ① ②
14. Impaired relationships .... ① ②
15. Impaired social performance (school/job) .... ① ②
16. Judgment/Informed Consent/AMA .... ① ②
17. Organic brain syndrome .... ① ②
18. Pain .... ① ②
19. Paranoid behavior .... ① ②
20. Patient requested consult .... ① ②
21. Postpartum condition .... ① ②
22. Preoperative evaluation .... ① ②
23. Pretransfer evaluation (to another med/surg unit).......... ① ②
24. Psychiatric History-nonpsychotic (minor) .... ① ②
25. Psychiatric History-psychotic (major) .... ① ②
26. Psychotropic medication assessment .... ① ②
27. Noncompliant, i.e., refusing tests or treatment .... ① ②
28. Reproductive disorders .... ① ②
29. Sexual Issues .... ① ②
30. Sleeping disorder .... ① ②
31. Staff problems .... ① ②
32. Suicidal risk/attempt evaluation .... ① ②
33. Terminal illness .... ① ②
34. Transfer to a psychiatric unit .... ① ②
35. Other .... ① ②

MEDICAL DIAGNOSIS (ICD-9) AXIS III

AXIS   AXIS V   KARNOFSKY RATING SCALE (See Codes P.2)   GLOBAL PSYCH IMPAIR-MENT

	PRE	TERM	PRE	TERM

PLEASE DO NOT MARK IN THIS AREA

RECOMMENDATIONS AND STATUS		
For each of the following indicate if you recommended:	ADDITIONAL LABORATORY TESTS (i.e., E.E.G., blood, etc.)	⓪ ⊕ ⊖ ① ② ③ ④ ⑤
	PSYCHOMETRIC TESTS (neuropsychiatric, affective, personality)	⓪ ⊕ ⊖ ① ② ③ ④ ⑤
0 = NO RECOMMENDATION MADE	ADDITIONAL MEDICAL / SURGICAL CONSULTATIONS	⓪ ⊕ ⊖ ① ② ③ ④ ⑤
+ = AN INCREASE OR ACCELERATION	NON-MEDICAL CONSULTATIONS (physical rehab, dietary, Social Work)	⓪ ⊕ ⊖ ① ② ③ ④ ⑤
- = DECREASE OR DELAY	GET INFORMATION FROM EXTERNAL SOURCES (family, friends, clinics, practitioners)	⓪ ⊕ ⊖ ① ② ③ ④ ⑤
Also at termination, indicate if each was:	INFLUENCE IMPLEMENTATION OF MEDICAL TREATMENT (VIGOR)	⓪ ⊕ ⊖ ① ② ③ ④ ⑤
	BEHAVIOR MANAGEMENT (restrain/activate/mobilize)	⓪ ⊕ ⊖ ① ② ③ ④ ⑤
1 = not performed	PSYCHOLOGICAL MANAGEMENT (educate/orient the patient/ psychotherapy/character management)	⓪ ⊕ ⊖ ① ② ③ ④ ⑤
2 = performed by consultant	ENVIRONMENTAL MANIPULATION (change location on unit, amount of patient contacts, observation)	⓪ ⊕ ⊖ ① ② ③ ④ ⑤
3 = performed by ward staff	SOCIAL SUPPORT...RELATIONSHIP WITH FAMILY, FRIENDS (arrange visits, educate/counsel family, include family in management)	⓪ ⊕ ⊖ ① ② ③ ④ ⑤
4 = performed by both or others	INFLUENCE DISCHARGE DATE (accelerate, delay, plan)	⓪ ⊕ ⊖ ① ② ③ ④ ⑤
5 = status unknown	AFTERCARE REFERRALS (with outpatient center, inpatient unit or physician)	⓪ ⊕ ⊖ ① ② ③ ④ ⑤

ADMINISTRATIVE ACTION	NUMBER OF FOLLOW UPS	PSYCHOTROPIC MEDICATION RECOMMENDED, STATUS AND ADVERSE REACTIONS

INFORMED CONSENT
① Patient is able to give informed consent
② Patient is not able to give informed consent
③ Informed consent was not an issue

A.M.A. (against medical advice)
① Patient may leave A.M.A.
② Patient may not leave A.M.A.
③ Patient leaving A.M.A. not an issue

INVOLUNTARY TRANSFER TO PSYCHIATRIC FACILITY
① Patient to be transferred involuntarily
② Involuntary transfer requested, but not appropriate
③ Involuntary transfer was not an issue

NUMBER OF FOLLOW UPS: ⓪ ⓪ / ① ① / ② ② / ③ ③ / ④ ④ / ⑤ ⑤ / ⑥ ⑥ / ⑦ ⑦ / ⑧ ⑧ / ⑨ ⑨

DRUG 1			DRUG 2		
CODE	STATUS	REACT	CODE	STATUS	REACT
⓪ ⓪ ⓪			⓪ ⓪ ⓪		
① ① ①	①	①	① ① ①	①	①
② ② ②	②	②	② ② ②	②	②
③ ③ ③	③	③	③ ③ ③	③	③
④ ④ ④	④	④	④ ④ ④	④	④
⑤ ⑤ ⑤	⑤	⑤	⑤ ⑤ ⑤	⑤	⑤
⑥ ⑥ ⑥	⑥	⑥	⑥ ⑥ ⑥	⑥	⑥
⑦ ⑦ ⑦	⑦	⑦	⑦ ⑦ ⑦	⑦	⑦
⑧ ⑧ ⑧			⑧ ⑧ ⑧		
⑨ ⑨ ⑨			⑨ ⑨ ⑨		

DISCHARGE LOCATION — Implemented / Recommended

	Rec	Impl
home	①	①
physical rehabilitation inpatient	②	②
somatic nursing home	③	③
psychiatric nursing home or residence	④	④
general hospital	⑤	⑤
psychiatric hospital	⑥	⑥
other institution	⑦	⑦
other living situation	⑧	⑧
unknown	⑨	⑨
does not apply	⑩	⑩

DRUG 3			DRUG 4		
CODE	STATUS	REACT	CODE	STATUS	REACT
⓪ ⓪ ⓪			⓪ ⓪ ⓪		
① ① ①	①	①	① ① ①	①	①
② ② ②	②	②	② ② ②	②	②
③ ③ ③	③	③	③ ③ ③	③	③
④ ④ ④	④	④	④ ④ ④	④	④
⑤ ⑤ ⑤	⑤	⑤	⑤ ⑤ ⑤	⑤	⑤
⑥ ⑥ ⑥	⑥	⑥	⑥ ⑥ ⑥	⑥	⑥
⑦ ⑦ ⑦	⑦	⑦	⑦ ⑦ ⑦	⑦	⑦
⑧ ⑧ ⑧			⑧ ⑧ ⑧		
⑨ ⑨ ⑨			⑨ ⑨ ⑨		

CONSULTATION TERMINATED BY:
① Psychiatric Consultant
② Transfer to private or other psychiatrist
③ Discharge with notice
④ Discharge without notice
⑤ Patient
⑥ Death
⑦ Administration
⑧ Admitted to psychiatric inpatient unit
⑨ Other

DATE CONSULTATION TERMINATED

M O	⓪ ①	⓪ ① ② ③ ④ ⑤ ⑥ ⑦ ⑧ ⑨
D A Y	⓪ ① ② ③	⓪ ① ② ③ ④ ⑤ ⑥ ⑦ ⑧ ⑨
Y R	⑧ ⑨	⓪ ① ② ③ ④ ⑤ ⑥ ⑦ ⑧ ⑨

DATE PATIENT DISCHARGED FROM HOSPITAL

M O	⓪ ①	⓪ ① ② ③ ④ ⑤ ⑥ ⑦ ⑧ ⑨
D A Y	⓪ ① ② ③	⓪ ① ② ③ ④ ⑤ ⑥ ⑦ ⑧ ⑨
Y R	⑧ ⑨	⓪ ① ② ③ ④ ⑤ ⑥ ⑦ ⑧ ⑨

AVERAGE TIME PER FOLLOW-UP
① None
② < 15 mins
③ 15-30 mins
④ 31-60 mins
⑤ 61 + mins

SUPERVISION TIME WITH ATTENDING IN 15-MINUTE UNITS	Initial	⓪ ① ② ③ ④ ⑤ ⑥ ⑦ ⑧ ⑨
		⓪ ① ② ③ ④ ⑤ ⑥ ⑦ ⑧ ⑨
	Total	⓪ ① ② ③ ④ ⑤ ⑥ ⑦ ⑧ ⑨
		⓪ ① ② ③ ④ ⑤ ⑥ ⑦ ⑧ ⑨

PLEASE DO NOT MARK IN THIS AREA

090105

Printed in U.S.A.   NCS Trans-Optic® MP30-77046-32

9

Recommendations

While consultation-liaison psychiatrists should link their recommendations closely to explicitly stated clinical questions, consultants may also have to assess a range of factors that affect the relationship between the primary-care staff and the patient. The consultant should always address any signs or symptoms noted by the primary physician that point to specific psychiatric disorders—depressed mood, vegetative signs, anesthesia inconsistent with nerve distributions, or cognitive deficits. However, when the primary physician covertly expresses frustration, guilt, and annoyance because he or she is unable to diagnose (Saravay and Koran 1977), treat, and discharge the patient from the hospital, the consultant's recommendations should also encompass those expressions. In such cases, the primary physician may request a consultation for reasons which mask his or her desire that the psychiatrist resolve the problem by arbitrating, counseling, or granting absolution for the patient (Krakowski 1979). Ultimately, consultants intervene in order to improve both the understanding and the working relationship between primary physician and patient so that diagnosis and therapy proceed effectively.

LIAISON

How you, as consultant, understand and work with the consulting service determines both what courses of action you recommend and how you communicate those recommendations. Because your recommendations may require that the consultee service carry out your instructions, you must determine whether the service can play its part effectively. For example, a very active surgical service is unlikely to be able to work with a consulting psychiatrist to establish a token economy that selectively reinforces certain healthy behaviors and punishes unhealthy or disruptive ones. In contrast, a pediatric ward might easily set up such a program. Thus, you must understand what the service can and will do in order to make realistic recommendations about patient care.

Because most patient treatments are handled in the short term, the consultant needs to decide who should initiate certain treatments and where these treatments should be initiated. For example, depressed medical inpatients may not need to be treated with antidepressant medications while they are in the general hospital, especially if they will soon be transferred to the care of another psychiatrist. While consultant and primary physician want to alleviate the patient's depression quickly, they must recognize that their intervention might prevent the follow-up psychiatrist from observing the patient's baseline presentation, choosing the medications with which he or she is most comfortable, and assessing the patient's responses to brief or cognitive interventions before initiating pharmacological treatments. On the other hand, the consultant might recommend early pharmacological intervention because he or she believes that alleviating biological symptoms will allow the follow-up psychiatrist to focus more rapidly on dynamic issues in the patient's disorder. Similarly, the consultant to a cardiology ward may recommend that a depressed patient with cardiac dysrhythmia or conduction defects be medicated immediately so that the doctor can assess whether the medication worsens the cardiac disorder. A medical-psychiatric ward or medical ward is probably the safest location for this sort of therapeutic trial. In making recommendations, the consultant also needs to determine when and where certain treatments should be initiated.

Consultation-liaison psychiatrists have to respond to other practical realities when they recommend initiating a psychiatric treatment. For example, if the service is unfamiliar with the timing necessary for obtaining accurate lithium blood levels, you may have to educate staff and ancillary personnel. You must advise the service of the possible short- and long-term extrapyramidal reactions of neuroleptic medication, the anticholinergic side effects of antidepressants, and the danger of using epinephrine with neuroleptic antipsychotic medication. The psychiatric consultant cannot manage treatment unless the service can absorb and use the information it is given.

Realistically, the psychiatric consultant cannot recommend appropriate treatments unless he or she understands how well hospital staff members relate to their patients who display psychopathology. Because the psychiatric consultation should help a medical staff and a patient work together to treat the patient's medical problems, consultant recommendations can arbitrate a give and take between patient and staff that enables them to work effectively together. For example, we were asked by the surgical service to consult on a patient who was refusing a gallbladder operation. The surgeons were upset when the patient refused the operation, and they insisted that he either be declared incompetent or transferred to the psychiatric hospital. An elderly, relatively unsophisticated gentleman, whose father had died during an operation, the patient was terrified that he too would die during the operation. With the consultant's mediation, the patient and surgeons were able to conservatively treat the problem with antibiotics and intravenous hydration on the condition that the patient accept the operation if the treatment trial failed. At times like this, recommendations need to be offered in a fashion both the service and the patient can accept.

When necessary, the consultant's recommendations should reflect his or her inability to easily diagnose and/or control certain situations. The consultant who can say "I don't know" at the appropriate time demonstrates professional maturity. In addition, a consultant who recommends continued structured observations, further diagnostic tests, or other consultation provides an appropriate role model for physicians in general, encouraging them to avoid premature conclusions about the patient's condition. Such recommendations also help the consultee deal with the reality that all symptoms in medical patients may have "functional" components. Through such recommendations, the consultant conveys the message that functional symptoms should be diagnosed by discrete criteria, rather than by simply excluding the most apparent medical differential diagnoses. The physician with an open mind is far less likely to misdiagnose the depressed patient with appendicitis or cancer. When the psychiatrist openly admits diagnostic uncertainty, he or she registers a welcome empathy with the primary physician who feels frustrated, guilty, and annoyed. Recommendations that take into account the difficulties of diagnosis embody the truth that these problems *are* frustrating, guilt-provoking, and annoying.

Types of Recommendations

We have divided recommendations into several categories that we consider useful. Our recommendation categories reflect a medical approach to psychiatric treatment that is particularly useful and collegial in the general-hospital setting.

Further Diagnostic Workup

Psychiatric Workup.   While many consultations may be effectively performed with the limited information available at the time of initial interview, a consultant may recognize that he or she cannot recommend treatment without knowing more about the patient. Of course, the consultant needs to tailor requests for observations to how psychologically sophisticated the medical team is and how complex the information is that he or she needs. At one end of the spectrum, requesting that a staff document crying spells, sleep patterns, and eating habits is relatively simple and often helpful to achieve a reliable diagnosis, for example, of affective disorders. By contrast, asking a staff to assess how a patient responds to increased social contact with hospital volunteers or physical therapists may require that the staff perform more sophisticated observations. Even diagnostic procedures guided by the psychiatrist, such as a trial of stimulants for psychomotorically retarded, medically ill elderly patients, and critical to managing patients who are difficult to ambulate and/or motivate, depend for their success on the appropriate feedback from the staff members who interact most with the patient.

Although a staff can supply a great deal of information, the consultant may also need to either perform some diagnostic procedures, such as an Amytal or hypnosis-aided interview, or a diagnostic biofeedback session on the medical floor, or initiate a brief treatment trial.

Consultations: Neuropsychological and Psychological Testing. Where time is limited, diagnostic evaluation in the medical setting can be supplemented by psychological tests. For example, the consultant might recommend such easily administered tests for bedbound patients as the Minnesota Multiphasic Personality Inventory (MMPI) for verification of depression, mania, factitious illness, somatization, etc. Other neuropsychological batteries, such as the Halstead-Reitan (Reitan and Davison 1974) and the Wechsler Adult Intelligence Scale—Revised (WAIS-R) (Wechsler 1981), might require that the patient be transported from the ward to the psychology department.

Because these tests quantify the degree of cognitive impairment suggested by simpler, interview-based tests (such as the Folstein-McHugh Mini-Mental State Exam [Folstein et al. 1975]), they often provide a useful baseline against which future deterioration or improvement in such function can be tested. Because the primary medical service generally has the authority to order further consultations, the psychiatric consultant must work with the medical team and the consulting psychologist to identify the types of tests, or more importantly, the type of information desired by the consultant. Ideally, the psychiatric consultant should talk directly with the psychologist in order to focus the psychological investigation.

Consultations: Medical and Neurological. In many cases, psychiatric diagnosis requires further diagnostic workup by medical specialists other than the primary medical service. Typically, the consultant may be unable to recommend a treatment until he or she sees the results of other specialty (e.g., neurologic, cardiac, gastroenterologic) evaluations.

For example, neurological consultants are essential to the detailed workup of patients who experience new onset dementias, seizure-like syndromes, headache, and neuropathy. Similarly, in order to evaluate psychophysiological and psychosomatic contributions to the complaint of chest pain, the consultant may also recommend specialized gastroenterologic evaluation using, for example, esophageal manometry, endoscopy, or assessments of nighttime acid reflux.

Because further requests for medical workups may offend the medical team to the degree that they refuse the consultant's recommendations, the consultant needs to address possible resistance directly and openly. In order to develop a working alliance with the physician, the consultant educates the primary physician about why the psychiatric diagnosis requires such specialized examinations and consultations—an understanding difficult to attain if consultant and consultee physician communicate only through the medical chart. Unless the psychiatrist documents why specific differential diagnostic questions need to be answered, he or she cannot identify the medical importance of the investigation.

Medical Workup: Laboratory Tests. Some psychiatric diagnoses will also require laboratory tests such as blood counts, electrolytes, endocrine function tests, microbiological cultures, or specific procedures such as electroencephalograms (EEGs), brain scans, or electromyograms (EMGs). In such cases, the consultant's recommendations can teach about how disease states affect mental status; they demonstrate your (medical) focus on the whole human being. Through recommendations you can show, for example, how organic brain syndromes and general symptoms of fatigue or irritability are associated with a variety of medical illnesses, particularly those illnesses that affect the CNS. Or you may suggest tests that demonstrate that symptoms of mood and/or anxiety disorders may result from thyroid dysfunction, brain injury, or pheochromocytomas, and are significant components of the differential diagnosis.

Medical Workup: Differential Diagnosis. Because a wide spectrum of disease processes, medical treatments, and substance abuses affect cognitive and affective states, psychiatrists will work closely with the nonpsychiatric physicians and consultants. Through such alliance, the psychiatric consultant can show the nonpsychiatric team how therapy choices are complicated by secondary affective symptoms resulting from steroid use, the toxic delirious state caused by digitalis, and the cholinergic psychosis that can result when antispasmodics and antidepressants are combined. Equally often, the consultant can elucidate the medical side effects of psychotropic drugs—the arrhythmogenic effects of antidepressants, the hypotensive effects of phenothiazines, and the CNS-sedating effects of benzodiazepines—and suggest why those drugs should not be given to medically ill patients.

Finally, primary physicians sometimes mislabel problems related to the patient's general condition as psychological. The primary physician may attribute malaise and weakness to depression rather than to a concurrent anemia, malnourished state, or other chronic disease. Consultant recommendations often focus on such general medical issues in order to determine whether or not a patient can live independently. In the same way, the consultant must consider diagnostic issues such as the patient's prognosis, capacity to perform activities of daily living, and ability to self-administer medical treatments (such as insulin in the case of the diabetic patient), before he or she completes a psychiatric assessment.

Consultations: Nonmedical. For these and other reasons, the psychiatric consultant may recommend other, nonmedical consultations to the team. These consultations are generally more common and numerous than recommendations for medical consultations. As before, the consultant must work closely with the primary physician to ensure that the consultant's or patient's needs are effectively translated into a consultation request. Such requests might include dietary assessment in the case of a brittle diabetic, physical therapy in the case of a marginally mobile stroke patient, or social work in the case of the homeless or destitute patient.

In fact, recommendations for social assessments are an essential ingredient in the evaluation of most consultation cases. Unlike office-based psychiatrists, consultation psychiatrists commonly ask family and significant others to independently assess hospitalized patients. In the medical hospital, patients are often too ill to give an adequate history. Sometimes these patients confabulate or have factitious illnesses, and thus cannot respond truthfully when asked about their own history. Because medically ill patients require a great deal of family involvement—both physical and emotional—the consultant needs to know whether the patient can depend on family support, particularly when that support could affect the safety of the patient or others. In some instances, information about the family's emotional and physical support might be gathered by the consultant; in other cases, it might be gathered by the medical team or social worker.

Behavior Management

Provisions for Patient Safety. Patient safety is the most important consideration in the management of all psychiatric (as well as medical) patients. However, while the Joint Commission on Accreditation of Hospitals (1988, p. 212) requires that hospital procedure manuals include specific guidelines for patients, most medical hospitals are not designed to provide a safe setting for psychiatric patients. Many medical wards do not have windows with grates, locks, or a centrally located nursing area to provide optimal observation. Consequently, consultants may need to outline the precautions the staff should take in order to treat certain patients safely.

To ensure that they do not harm themselves, acutely suicidal or delirious patients are generally assigned one-to-one, around-the-clock supervision. Preferably, the "sitter" should be an experienced psychiatric nurse. Given the current shortage of registered nurses, however, sitters are often untrained nursing assistants. Therefore, either the psychiatric consultant or psychiatrically trained nurses should ensure that sitters are properly prepared to deal with potentially dangerous patients.

The consultant should see that the sitter is provided with written, detailed instructions (see Appendix) explaining how to observe suicidal patients. Ideally, these instructions tell the sitter how to supervise the patient while the latter is using sharp objects, glassware, eating utensils, needles, razor blades, matches, and belts. The sitter should also be told to continue one-to-one supervision when the patient is smoking or passes through dangerous areas on the medical floor, such as balcony areas or rooms that contain poisons or have windows open. If possible, the patient's activity should be limited to the ward. When leaving the ward for a medical test, the patient must be accompanied by the sitter. Nursing staff should monitor the patient's visitors to ensure that they do not leave the patient potentially harmful objects. The sitter must be instructed to maintain close proximity to the patient at all times, even while the patient is bathing or using the toilet. As primary observers, sitters must also be specifically instructed to have someone else monitor the patient whenever they need to leave the patient, even if briefly, to eat or to go to the bathroom.

Just as important, the consultant can help sitters understand that they play a key role in documenting any unusual or suspicious statements, behaviors, and/or mood changes. With proper instructions, these relatively untrained people can be excellent resources for direct, continuous observations of the patient's behavior. The consultant should work with the sitter to generate a list of specific behaviors or physiological patterns to be identified and tallied, such as crying, sleeping, eating, reading, and how the patient receives visitors. As in the psychiatric hospital, the consultant uses the patient's clinical condition to determine when to discontinue the sitter. As the clinical condition improves, a step-down level of observation, such as close observations—that is eye contact every 15 minutes of the patient who is limited to the floor—can be used. The consultant can work with the staff to monitor this stepping down, to decide when a recovering patient can, for example, be moved to a bed nearer to the nursing station for less constant, but steady, observation by the nurses.

Restraints. While proper observation contributes to safety, medical wards require such further safety measures as bed bars, separation from other patients, and restraints. Sometimes, wards may even need a group of strong aides who can physically subdue the acutely agitated patient. When patients who are potentially violent are hospitalized, the nursing staff should obtain the names, locations, and phone numbers of nursing assistants working on other wards who may be summoned on short notice to provide assistance. In some hospitals, the staff may also use police or security guards to help them handle difficult patients. However, police or security guard personnel are less desirable than nursing assistants unless the former have been trained to manage violence in medically ill or psychiatrically disturbed individuals. In making patient recommendations, the consultation-liaison psychiatrist thus must be aware of the extent to which the staff are capable of handling disruptive and/or dangerous patients.

While physical restraints can save lives on medical wards, the staff must know when to use restraints so that they can avoid untoward reactions by the patient. Restraints are appropriate for a range of situations including psychotic agitation and various agitations or confusions associated with acute and chronic organic brain syndromes; however, staff must never use restraints to "punish" patients for bad behavior. Despite this limit on physical restraints, potentially dangerous patients must be behaviorally managed to protect staff and other patients, and because patients and staff have successfully sued other patients for assault, even in the case of nonpsychotic patients on psychiatric wards (Phelan et al. 1985).

Thus, the consultant can work with the staff to see that physical restraints are used appropriately and effectively. The hospital procedure manual should publish specific guidelines for how to use physical restraints, guidelines that reflect statutory mandates that the patient be cared for in the least restrictive environment. Provide a copy of the guidelines to the medical service or sitter. Staff must also be instructed to intermittently remove the restraints, to test for overtightness, and to frequently observe the patient both day and night to avoid injury or further agitation. Even under restraint, the patient must be able to move around enough to avoid decubitus sores or atelectasis. We further recommend that restraints not be applied to only the upper or lower extremities, because this form of restraint increases the possibility that patients will injure themselves if they attempt to leave their beds. The nurse assigned to care for the restrained patient often can recommend when the restraint can be removed. Finally, both consultant and staff should be aware that removing restraints from a patient with frightening and unpredictable behavior raises the level of anxiety on the medical/surgical floor.

In many circumstances, chemical or social restraints are safe and effective alternatives to physical restraint. Physical restraint may, for example, increase agitation and exacerbate cardiac or pulmonary symptoms in some patients. Conversely, the interaction of tranquilizers and medical illness or other medications makes chemical restraint unsafe in certain patients.

However, the extent of behavioral disturbance can limit the

effectiveness of social restraint. Consider a patient on the orthopedic surgery ward with osteomyelitis whose secret drinking drives him to such aggressive activities as destroying the patient phone box, throwing trays, and verbally abusing the staff. In the patient's baseline state, his behavior was not perfect, but he was calm and cooperative. While he was drunk, his behavior was disruptive and dangerous. At last, the hospital staff's anxiety became so great that the hospital sought legal counsel to forcibly discharge the patient before he had finished the requisite course of intravenously administered antibiotics. During a period of calm, the patient was apprised of the impending discharge and how it would affect his well-being. He agreed to stay off alcohol and, more importantly, to begin taking disulfiram (to allay staff fears about his reliability). In this case, social restraints resolved the situation.

Monitoring of Visitors. Psychiatric consultation can also help the medical-ward staff deal with disruptions associated with visitors. For example, medical staff may find it difficult to monitor visitors who bring in substances (such as drugs or alcohol) that can adversely affect a patient when that patient is not hospitalized for detoxification. The patient may view hospitalization as serving the sole purpose of curing a chest pain (myocarditis), an infection, or an injury; thus, he or she might experience detoxification from drugs or alcohol as an unreasonable intrusion. Indeed, the boredom of hospitalization can make drug or alcohol use even more attractive to such patients. Despite these difficulties, drug-induced alterations in behavior disrupt medical wards and need to be controlled. The staff may need to use blood/urine toxicology to screen suspect patients. Ideally, the staff should openly address the intoxicated behavior and tell the patient that they intend to test for street drugs. Although most patients sign a blanket consent for laboratory tests related to their medical condition (except for the AIDS virus), surreptitious tests indicate that the doctor-patient relationship lacks the mutual respect essential for effective medical treatment. In any case, negative tests often assure the staff, who are generally more comfortable dealing with the chaotic behavior that results from psychiatric disturbance than with the chaotic behavior that results from drug abuse.

The psychiatric consultant can also guide or advise the staff that needs to monitor visitors for other reasons. Even more frustrating, visitors may be disruptive or too stimulating for the patient. Their behavior may adversely affect other patients or their visitors. Visitors also may prevent the medical and/or nonmedical staff from effectively carrying out their duties. In any of these cases, the staff might need to restrict visitation. To help the staff cope with these difficulties, the consultant should encourage the staff to extensively document the specific behaviors of patient and visitors and how those behaviors interfere with the functioning of the medical team and the progress of other patients' treatment. The consultant may also seek guidance from hospital attorneys when recommending restricted visitation or other potentially incitive measures.

Discharge Against Medical Advice. The psychiatric consultant is often emergently called to evaluate the competence of patients who wish to leave the hospital against medical advice (designated AMA). If the consultant finds that such a patient meets the criteria for civil commitment, he or she may hold the patient for psychiatric treatment.

Patients may want to leave against medical advice for a variety of reasons. Sometimes, the patient uses the AMA designation to deny the seriousness of the medical situation. Such patterns of denial are common in coronary care units in postmyocardial infarction patients (Cassem and Hackett 1987). Delirious, demented, and paranoid patients may want to leave against medical advice because they are confused about the motives of the health-care providers. Other patients are angry at the staff, accusing them of inconsiderate or brusque treatment. In some cases, disagreement about proposed interventions may be a factor. The consultant needs to be aware that each situation requires different strategies. In the case of the demented or paranoid patient who refuses treatment, for example, the patient's capacity to provide informed consent may be at issue. The consultant must soothe the narcissistic injuries suffered by both the patient and the treating physician, and attempt to improve the empathic understanding between them. In cases where the patient refuses certain treatments (such as surgery or biopsy) and the medical staff refuses to provide the patient with *any* alternatives, the consultant should seek to foster compromise solutions.

While it is often difficult to identify the specific transactions between staff and patient that trigger the patient's attempt to leave the hospital against medical advice, how the consultant assesses whether to allow a patient to leave in this way is conceptually straightforward. Basically, the consultant must determine whether that patient meets the criteria for civil commitment set out in state guidelines. According to California and Illinois, the patient must be found to be a danger to self, a danger to others, or gravely disabled by virtue of a mental disorder. If the patient meets these criteria, then he or she may be held against his or her will for psychiatric treatment. Thus, the consultant may use this procedure to prevent the patient from leaving the hospital against medical advice.

In order to deal effectively with AMA problems, the consultant should become familiar with the statutory rules in the state in which he or she practices. Because some states specifically restrict the commitment of psychiatric patients to wards in psychiatric hospitals, consultants may need legal counsel about the requirements of a particular state's commitment laws.

Consent to Treatment. Once committed, if the (competent) patient agrees to receive psychiatric or medical treatment, treatment commences. Psychiatric commitments can only be instituted on patients for purposes of psychiatric treatment—not medical treatment. With the exception of *emergency* psychiatric treatment in certain states, however, committing the patient to the hospital does not mean that the patient can be treated with any medication or procedure against his or her will.

Once the patient has been committed, the consultant must then ascertain whether the patient has the "capacity" to understand the nature of the treatment proposed and the risks and benefits of the treatment, of nontreatment, or of alternative treatments. While this determination is commonly referred to as "competency to consent to treatment," competency is a *legal* determination performed by judges rather than psychiatrists. Nevertheless, judges rely on the expert opinion of psychiatrists as to whether the patient has the capacity to consent. Called in by the court, the psychiatrist provides an opinion as to whether the patient can understand issues related to treatment. A patient may, for example, be demented but still adequately understand the treatment recommended and the alternatives available. Sometimes, a patient's perceived "incompetence" results from information ineffectively communicated. In such situations, the psychiatrist may need to discuss in detail the elements of the proposed treatment with the patient.

When an intervention must be performed immediately in order to avoid irreversible injury, the consultant must know that emergency treatment is handled differently than commitment. For example, California and Illinois require two signatures by licensed physicians to institute emergency treatment. In contrast, nonemergent treatment for patients who are unable to provide consent often requires court approval. Some jurisdictions allow a close family member to provide substituted consent, particularly for minor procedures such as spinal tap. Recent legislative changes have made it possible for a patient to assign a family member or friend the power to make medical decisions for the patient in the event that he or she becomes unable to provide informed consent. In California, this prior assignment is called a "Durable Power of Attorney for Health Care": the patient is called the "principal," and the family member or friend making the substituted consent is designated the "attorney in fact." The Durable Power of Attorney requires the physician to follow the treatment decisions of the substituted consenter or attorney in fact, except in specifically delineated circumstances, such as when the principal has revoked the durable power of attorney. Given these legislative differences, the consultant should work with the hospital's attorney to familiarize himself or herself with local regulations governing involuntary treatment and substituted consent.

Discharge and Dangerousness.   Dangerous or suicidal patients present the consultation-liaison psychiatrist with different medical and legal problems. In dangerous-to-others (DTO) cases, the consultant may be involved in determining the degree to which the patients are dangerous to others, in providing a safe environment for initial interventions, in managing interventions, and in warning individuals and agencies when a patient is dangerous.

Dangerousness to others is a heterogeneous, nonspecific set of complex behaviors that may reflect varying DSM-III-R diagnoses, including organic brain syndromes, functional psychoses, epilepsy, drug and alcohol abuse, personality disorders, or a combination of these diagnoses. As most psychiatrists know, the stress of medical hospitalization or illness may overpower a patient's ability to control such impulses. Thus, the consultant who works in a hospital setting may encounter patients who are anxious about their illness, do not understand either that illness or the hospital milieu, and are frustrated by the uncertainties of medical treatment—potential DTO cases. While nonpsychiatric staff and security officers have a duty to restrain a patient until the psychiatrist arrives in order to protect other patients from harm, in most jurisdictions, psychiatrists are the only professionals legally qualified and mandated to assess the degree to which patients are dangerous to others. As medical emergencies, DTO cases require immediate response on the part of the ward staff; they also require that a psychiatrist perform a complete assessment of the patient.

After assessing dangerousness to others, the consultant can see that the patient has a safe environment (until transferred to a suitable facility or ward) and may even manage or recommend interventions and further treatment. Generally, DTO patients will need to be managed on the medical/surgical floors until their medical condition allows them to be transferred to an appropriate psychiatric facility. During this period, the consultant may work with the staff to set up such appropriate interventions as interpersonal therapies to help buttress the patient's defenses, controls, and/or adaptation; pharmacotherapy to treat specific diagnostic problems; environmental changes, such as moving the patient to a private room; and restraints in the form of a sitter or physical restraint. During the initial intervention process, the consultant must also determine whether or not the patient meets criteria for involuntary certification.

After the acute episode (prior to discharge), the consultant must determine whether or not issuance of a *Tarasoff* warning is indicated. The *Tarasoff* decision stems from a California court ruling that established that psychiatrists have a duty to warn intended victims of violent assault by psychiatric patients (*Tarasoff* 1976). In many jurisdictions, this doctrine has been expanded to include warnings by nonpsychiatric therapists as well as warnings to potential victims (as opposed to definitely intended victims). In California, the legislature has recently limited liability for failure to warn specifically identifiable victims. Legally, however, the duty to protect a third person from foreseeable danger—a future act of violence against the third person—by a psychiatrist's patient outweighs the doctor's duty to maintain patient confidentiality.

Finally, the consultant must also remember to advise the primary-care physician of his or her duty to notify the appropriate agencies of patients who are indirectly dangerous. For example, the Department of Motor Vehicles must be notified of patients who are prone to blackouts, whether due to seizures, pseudoseizures, or syncope. Some health departments may need to be notified of certain infectious diseases, particularly when the consultant discovers that a patient intends to infect others either maliciously or because he or she is unable to properly notify potential victims. Psychiatrists are also frequently confronted with amnesic or demented patients whose forgetfulness could endanger many lives should they leave a burning cigarette or flaming stove in their apartment. In all cases, psychiatrists should maintain a record of warnings.

Treatment

Social Intervention. In collaboration with other appropriate members of the team (nurses, social workers, dietitians, psychologists), the psychiatric consultant can recommend many types of social interventions necessary to or helpful for the patient's recuperation. The consultant may choose to perform some interventions directly or may recommend that they be implemented by the primary-care team or another consulting service. This team approach not only facilitates the patient's needs but also ensures that the consultant's time is used effectively.

In hospital settings, social workers are particularly helpful because they can refer the patient and family to community resources that can buffer the effects of the patient's decreased physical abilities. This assistance may range from helping the patient obtain disability to helping a family member become conservator of a patient who is unable to provide for his or her own care. In turn, psychiatric involvement in conservatorship hearings or disability evaluations (Okpaku 1988) facilitates social workers' efforts to provide patient care. More generally, such ancillary services are financially important for hospitals because they reduce length of stay. To best serve both patient and hospital, psychiatric consultants need to be aware of the range of community resources, such as "meals on wheels," visiting nurses/home-based health services, housing services, and welfare assistance, that facilitate early discharge of patients who could not live independently without these support services.

The psychiatric consultant should encourage other social interventions. The nursing staff can help teach patients and/or family members about home medical treatment regimens, such as how to administer insulin or change bandages and how to document medical treatments to be performed by visiting nurses. The chaplain or minister can mobilize support from other church members. The primary medical team or occupational therapist can be called upon to explain the patient's condition and needs to his or her employers.

In addition, the consultant and the medical team should seek to involve the family in providing critical support for the patient. To foster this support, the consultant joins other team members in a family conference to identify the changes in family roles or the patient's aftercare needs. The team should guide members of a patient's family while the patient is still hospitalized. The family will better appreciate the patient's medical condition if they attend a family session with the consultant present. Such sessions are especially valuable when the patient develops a paranoid reaction in response to a medication, and the family mistrusts either the patient's intentions or his or her sanity. The consultant may also find family conferences valuable in cases such as that of the alcoholic patient with an amnestic syndrome who would like to return home to his family. Without family conferences that provide planned countermeasures, the patient might get lost, leave the stove or a cigarette burning, or be left alone for dangerously long periods of time.

In cases where patients leave against medical advice, while denying the seriousness of their illness, family involvement sometimes saves lives. The consultant can alert the family to signs or symptoms that indicate a deteriorating condition in the terrified patient. Often, the consultant and the medical team can involve the family in convincing a patient who wants to leave against medical advice to stay for the duration of his or her treatment. Social interventions can also involve people outside the patient's immediate family, such as attorneys, friends, and clergy.

The psychiatric consultant should make it a common practice to work with the primary-care service to involve the family or friends in a patient's management. Family members often feel intimidated by the hospital and its busy personnel, and are therefore reluctant to ask questions about their possible role in the aftercare of the patient. For this reason, the medical service must sometimes be encouraged to seek out and to educate the family about how the family members can help the patient recuperate. Commonly, a family member will need to administer the patient's medications or treatments. Sometimes, family and friends may need to help alter the patient's living environment—to install, for example, ramps for wheelchair access. The patient's return visits to the clinic might require the involvement of a dedicated and available family member. Whenever possible, then, the consultant should encourage the primary-care service to work with a patient's social support system; this interaction is often critical to effectively managing the patient's hospitalization and smooth discharge. While many patients find it difficult to ask their significant others for assistance, their mood and outlook on life is generally more positive when family or friends are involved in their aftercare.

Finally, a range of additional social factors affect the consultant's assessment, brief treatment, and discharge of patients with medical illnesses: Does the patient have friends? Does he or she have financial resources? Does the patient have a stable employment history? For example, the physically disabled, postmyocardial infarction patient who lives alone, has no immediate family, and has only worked as a stunt man will need both financial assistance and considerable help finding a new job. He might even require alternative temporary living arrangements before he can return to an apartment. By contrast, a similarly disabled, retired patient who lives with friends in a house, and has adequate retirement income, may have no difficulties going home after the acute hospitalization. The consultant who understands these social factors can make the most realistic and most successful recommendations.

Psychotherapeutic Treatment. Acute hospitalization variably represents a time of crisis, loss, impairment, and uncertainty; it may even restructure the patient's conception of himself or herself. Patients whose defenses have been weakened by illness or by separation from loved ones and home environment, as well as by the shock of being ill, need support and understanding. In this state, they are frequently unusually open to psychotherapeutic change. The psychiatric consultant should be familiar with the advantages and shortcomings of a wide variety of treatment options in order to focus a treatment plan—whether or not he or she will implement all or part of the patient's further treatment.

Acutely, the consultation-liaison psychiatrist's brief interventions, like those of the emergency-room psychiatrist, enhance the patient's weakened defenses in order to provide support and restore the premorbid level of psychological functioning. At this point, the consultation-liaison psychiatrist can identify acute stressors, determine usual coping strategies, and engage resources to help minimize the former and maximize the latter. Commonly, consultation-liaison psychiatrists implement brief treatments including psychodynamically based brief treatment (Davanloo 1980; Sifneos 1979), crisis intervention, cognitive therapy (Beck 1976), interpersonal therapy (Klerman 1984), and behavioral treatments (Garrick and Loewenstein 1989; Goldiamond 1979) such as cognitive therapy (Beck 1976), biofeedback (Olton and Noonberg 1980), systematic desensitization (Wolpe 1973), behavioral analysis (Fordyce and Steger 1979; Garrick 1981), and social skills training (Liberman et al. 1989). The consultant should tailor these brief treatments to the specific needs of the hospitalized patient.

Psychopharmacological Treatment. Psychoactive substances are the most prescribed medicines worldwide, and most of these prescriptions are written by nonpsychiatrists (Balter 1973). These medications produce staggeringly frequent side effects, which are even more common in medically compromised patients, because medical illness and organ failure can alter the normal excretion pathways and blood levels of psychotropic medications. Conversely, psychoactive medications can affect the course of medical illness: antidepressants have bundle branch–blocking properties, and neuroleptics lower the seizure threshold. As a class, geriatric patients are more sensitive to the effects and side effects of many medications. Thus, recommendations to alter dosage, obtain blood levels, and change medications must be explained in detail in the medical record.

Drug-drug interactions also result in iatrogenic complications, and as more and more medications are developed and used, these interactions increasingly complicate the physician's job. Often, the psychiatric consultant is in the position of trying to figure out which medication is causing a particularly disturbing side effect in the patient. For example, drugs that slow gastrointestinal transit enhance absorption of other orally administered drugs. Some medications may bind to other pharmacological agents, thus lowering their effective plasma level, as in the case of cholestyramine and the phenothiazines. Chloral hydrate and other psychoactive medications may bind to plasma proteins and displace other medications, such as warfarin, with medically disastrous results. Biotransformational alterations, such as the stimulation of hepatic microsomal enzyme by phenytoin, may decrease blood levels of other medicines such as phenobarbital.

In addition, various pharmacological agents may accentuate or antagonize each other's effects. The anticholinergic effects of a wide variety of medicines such as antispasmodics and analgesics can precipitate an anticholinergic psychosis or delirium if the patient is also receiving a tricyclic antidepressant. Adding two medications with enhancing pharmacological properties at different receptor sites can also be dangerous; thus, when phenothiazine medications, which are [alpha symbol]-receptor blockers, are combined with epinephrine, which has [beta symbol]-receptor–stimulating properties, the combined receptor actions can cause hypotension that is difficult to reverse.

Of course, the combined sedating properties of analgesics and tranquilizers are a frequent problem in medical patients. In postsurgical patients, drug-induced sedation is often a factor in postoperative delirium and may make it difficult to diagnose intraoperative complications such as hypoxic episodes. The hospital pharmacist can often provide information on these interactions as well as on idiosyncratic or unusual side effects.

In addition to making recommendations about doses and side effects, the psychiatric consultant should delineate the end points of treatment. Carefully delineated end points are particularly important when medications must be carefully titrated to specifically definable effects. For example, major tranquilizers are used to counter the effects of steroid-induced mania. Some medications, such as tricyclic antidepressants, must also be titrated to their side effects, such as anticholinergic symptoms. Because nonpsychiatric physicians are not generally well versed in psychotropic medication usage, the consultant should provide primary physicians with the specific information that will help ensure that the patient is properly medicated.

Special Referral. Hospitalization and medical illness strain the patient's coping mechanisms and may cause dysphoria, anxiety, and/or other psychiatric symptoms. Often, the consultation-liaison psychiatrist can identify specific resources and special services, available either in the hospital or privately, to assist the patient. Consultant referrals can have profound effects on the patient's mental well-being. For example, an ombudsman can help the patient negotiate confusing hospital bureaucracies, while a physical therapist can help the newly ambulatory patient feel confident about his or her ability to move about with or without special devices. Legal consultation or occupational therapy may alleviate problems caused by the patient's recent infirmity such as losing a business during prolonged hospitalization. Social work referral has a pivotal role in discharge planning, because illness may be worsened if patients are unable to adapt to their social environment and need help finding the alternative support that would allow them to live independently. In certain areas, special programs for patients with seizure disorder, amyotrophic lateral sclerosis, systemic lupus erythematosus, or inflammatory bowel disease, etc., may also be available.

Transfer and Referral. The psychiatric consultant's role is often pivotal in the transfer of patients to other facilities. In order to manage patient transfers, the consultant must know which institutions—for example, nursing homes—have restrictions on the kinds of behavioral disturbance they tolerate. Certain patients may require further inpatient treatment before they can be discharged to the community. Whereas some patients may need only a sheltered living arrangement such as a halfway

house or a board-and-care unit, other patients may require transfer to a medical psychiatric unit, an inpatient psychiatric unit, or
a state hospital. The consultant must recognize that he or she has
been called in to provide professional expertise in these areas.
The consultant assesses both the patient and the available facilities and then provides an appropriate referral.

Psychiatric Follow-up: Delineation of Responsibility. The
consultation-liaison psychiatrist has an unusual opportunity to
follow patients in a controlled medical environment. Psychiatric
follow-up is indicated in situations where intervention facilitates
medical recovery and discharge—for example, when the patient's
safety is compromised because of a psychiatric condition.
Through follow-ups, the consultant can help the patient with
psychological distress independent of the illness, or he or she can
help a medical staff work with a particular patient. In all circumstances, however, the consultant must coordinate follow-up with
the primary service so that staff members do not waste time
looking for patients off the floor for medical tests or treatments.
The psychiatric consultant should help allay staff anxiety about
the care of a disturbed patient. The consultant should document
in the chart the date, time, and place of follow-up appointments.
When he or she makes special referrals, these should be delineated in the record. At other times, the consultee service may
need to contact the consultant to coordinate treatments or transfers, impart information such as acute changes in status, or
request information that may be relevant to the medical treatment. The consultant may also wish to be notified if the patient
becomes more agitated, experiences a new onset of delirium,
recovers from sedation, or when the staff receives test results.
The consultant should spell out the specific danger signals (e.g.,
increase in command hallucinations) or worrisome side effects
(e.g., extrapyramidal neurological symptoms, unexpected sedation, cardiac dysrhythmia, or hypotension) that indicate that he
or she should be called.

To ensure maximum staff cooperation, the psychiatric consultant needs to specify the limits and end points of psychiatric
intervention. If the consultant requires that the primary-care
staff actively involve themselves in intervention, he or she must
explain the means and goals and see that the staff agrees with

them. If the consultant refers the patient to other psychiatrists or other health professionals, such as outpatient follow-up, or specialty programs, such as drug rehabilitation or pain clinic, he or she should also explain to the service and identify these changes in the medical record.

In conclusion, the consultant's recommendations define the breadth of the relationship between the psychiatric consultant, the consultee service, and the referred patient in terms of diagnosis, treatment, and disposition. The consultant must be explicit in the medical record when he or she suggests workups and determines who is responsible for doing workups, because recommendations involve all those people who handle additional workup, treatment, and disposition planning. Finally, the consultant should clearly identify, and coordinate with the primary medical service, those aspects of treatment recommendations he or she will perform.

REFERENCES

Balter MB: An analysis of psychotherapeutic drug consumption in the United States, in Proceedings of the Anglo-American Conference on Drug Abuse: Etiology of Drug Abuse, Vol 1. Edited by Bowen RA. London, Royal Society of Medicine, 1973, pp 58–65

Beck AT: Cognitive Therapy and the Emotional Disorders. New York, International Universities Press, 1976

Cassem NH, Hackett TP: The setting of intensive care, in Massachusetts General Hospital Handbook of General Hospital Psychiatry. Edited by Hackett TP, Cassem NH. Littleton, MA, PSG Publishers, 1987, pp 353–379

Davanloo H: Short-Term Dynamic Psychotherapy. New York, Jason Aronson, 1980

Folstein MF, Folstein SE, McHugh PR: Mini-Mental State: a practical method for grading the cognitive state of patients for the clinician. J Psychiatr Res 12:189–198, 1975

Fordyce WE, Steger JC: Chronic pain, in Behavioral Medicine: Theory and Practice. Edited by Pomerleau OF, Brady JP. Baltimore, MD, Williams & Wilkins, 1979, pp 125–153

Garrick T: Behavior therapy for irritable bowel syndrome. Gen Hosp Psychiatry 3:48–51, 1981

Garrick T, Loewenstein R: Behavioral medicine in the general hospital. Psychosomatics 30:123–134, 1989

Goldiamond I: Behavioral approaches and liaison psychiatry. Psychiatr Clin North Am 2:379–401, 1979

Joint Commission on Accreditation of Hospitals: Accreditation Manual for Hospitals. Chicago, IL, Joint Commission on Accreditation of Hospitals, 1988

Klerman GL, Weisman MM, Rounsaville BJ, et al: Interpersonal Psychotherapy of Depression. New York, Basic Books, 1984

Krakowski AJ: Liaison psychiatry in the West: the view from 1977. Psychother Psychosom 31:98–105, 1979

Liberman RP, DeRisi WJ, Mueser KT: Social Skills Training for Psychiatric Patients. New York, Pergamon, 1989

Okpaku SO: The psychiatrist and the social security disability insurance and supplemental security income programs. Hosp Community Psychiatry 39:879–883, 1988

Olton DS, Noonberg AR: Biofeedback: Clinical Applications in Behavioral Medicine. Englewood Cliffs, NJ, Prentice-Hall, 1980

Phelan LA, Mills MJ, Ryan JA: Prosecuting psychiatric patients for assault. Hosp Community Psychiatry 36:581–582, 1985

Reitan RM, Davison LA (eds): Clinical Neuropsychology: Current Status and Applications. Washington DC, Winston and Sons, 1974

Saravay SM, Koran LM: Organic disease mistakenly diagnosed as psychiatric. Psychosomatics 18:6–11, 1977

Sifneos PE: Short-Term Dynamic Psychotherapy Evaluation and Technique. New York, Plenum, 1979

Tarasoff v Regents of the University of California, 131 Cal Rptr 14 (1976)

Wechsler D: Wechsler Adult Intelligence Scale-Revised. New York, Psychological Corporation, 1981

Wolpe J: The Practice of Behavior Therapy. New York, Pergamon, 1973

APPENDIX: SAMPLE BRIEFING SHEET FOR NURSING ASSISTANTS ASSIGNED TO MONITOR SUICIDAL PATIENTS

SUICIDAL PRECAUTIONS

Close Observation Status and Suicidal Status

I. *IMPORTANT CONSIDERATIONS*

A. Suicidal precautions require either *Close Observation Status* or *Suicidal Status* and must be so specified. A patient may be placed on Suicidal ("S") Status by the admitting physician, ward physician, professional nurse, Mental Health Clinical Nurse Specialist, and/or consulting psychiatrist. When, in the opinion of the primary physician, the patient no longer requires suicidal precautions, the patient must be seen and reevaluated by a psychiatrist or psychiatric resident, and a written recommendation to remove the patient from suicidal precautions is to be provided in the progress notes.

B. The Nursing Supervisor is to be notified, and the patient's Medical Doctor is to contact the Psychiatric Evaluation and Admissions Unit.

C. Suicides are most common in the early morning hours, when the shift changes, and on or around holidays.

D. The following are symptoms of depression and may, especially in combination, be danger signs for suicidal behavior indicative of suicidal risk:

1. Early morning wakening and difficulty in falling asleep and/or staying asleep
2. Extreme slowing down of activity or extreme agitation
3. Decrease or increase in appetite
4. Sudden, unexplained mood changes
5. Isolative, morose behavior
6. Decreased attention to personal appearance

E. Schizophrenic patients who are having auditory hallucinations are particularly at risk for suicide if the voices are telling them to harm themselves or that it is time to die.

F. Suicidal patients are asking for help. Often they are ambivalent and cannot communicate their pain. They may wish to be saved from their own self-destructive impulses. The suicidal patient may be sending these messages

1. Make things better for me.
2. Help me control myself before I do some damage.
3. Help me!
4. Listen to me!

G. Note in the patient-care plan any predisposing factors taken from the patient's history (e.g., family history of suicidal behavior).

H. Factors such as a suicide plan, feelings of hopelessness, and previous suicidal behavior increase the risk for suicide.

II. *NURSING INTERVENTIONS*

A. *Close Observation Status*

1. Provide physical safety (see Suicidal Status).
2. If possible, have the patient in a room close to the nursing station, with alert patients, and where the patient is as visible as possible.
3. Assign the same nursing staff person as much as possible to care for the potentially suicidal patient and to help improve communication.
4. Report any unusual or suspicious statements (e.g., "I may not be here much longer") and/or mood changes to the charge nurse immediately. Mood changes, including what seem to be improvements, may actually indicate increased lethality.
5. Make pertinent nursing notes on each tour of duty.

B. *Suicidal Status*

1. A specially assigned (one-to-one) nurse is required for an acutely suicidal or potentially lethal patient. This

nurse is required to read the Suicidal Precautions Procedure and should be familiar with the hospital policy.

2. Provide physical safety

   a. Supervise use of sharp objects, glassware, eating utensils, smoking materials, needles, razor blades, poisons, matches, belts, bathing area, and areas of hazard on the unit such as those near balconies or open windows.

   b. Inspect patient's bedside cabinet and locker for the above items, remove if necessary, and tell the patient why.

   c. Limit the patient's activity to the ward, or always accompany the patient when he or she must go off the ward.

   d. Monitor the patient's visitors to ensure that they do not leave the patient any potentially harmful objects.

   e. Use protective restraints as a last resort (see policy).

3. Nursing personnel is to stay within close proximity of the patient at all times, even when the patient is bathing or using the toilet.

4. If possible, place the patient in a room with alert patients, close to the nursing station, and where they are always observed by nursing personnel.

5. Report any unusual or suspicious statements, behaviors, and/or mood changes to the charge nurse immediately (see Close Observation Status).

6. If a suicidal patient is to be transferred to the acute psychiatric facility for admission and/or evaluation, he or she is to be escorted by a nursing staff member. The nursing staff member is to remain with the patient until the disposition is made.

C. Contact the Mental Health Clinical Nurse Specialist whenever there is a concern or questions about the patient's status or the nursing interventions currently being utilized.

10

Follow-Through, Follow-Up, and Closing the Consultation

Failure to follow through and follow up are major complaints of primary physicians about psychiatric consultation and constitute a clinical failure in the care of the patient. Conversely, ongoing involvement in clinical assessment demonstrates, in the most useful and memorable way, the consultant's interest, availability, knowledge, skill, and sense of collaboration (Karasu et al. 1977). Follow-up must be reasoned and planned (Lipowski 1974), and the plans must be shared with, and accepted by, both the consultee and the patient. Follow-up must be carried out as planned unless the reasons for any changes are again explained and accepted.

It is vital that all follow-up efforts, including contacts with the patient, discussions with others involved with the case, relevant literature review, and even unsuccessful attempts to accomplish any of these, be documented in the chart (Garrick and Stotland 1982). In the perception of the primary service, and of the law, generally speaking, what is unrecorded never happened. But communication should not be limited to entries in the chart. Face-to-face and telephone interactions with the primary service are also important.

ASSESSING THE NEED FOR FOLLOW-UP

Every consultation case does not require follow-up. What is necessary is to make a considered, documented, and acceptable decision. When you have formulated the case, and as you are preparing to talk to the staff and write the formal consultation note, consider whether the primary physician's consultation question has been answered. For example, is the patient "paranoid" or "depressed" or "suicidal," as was suspected? Is the mental status change secondary to steroid administration, or schizophrenia?

The consultation question may have been in the form of a clinical problem, such as "bizarre behavior," "noncompliant with treatment," or "refuses to sign for surgery—please advise as to competency." In any case, the consultant must try to figure out both what the consultee is asking and what might help the consultee and the patient (Schiff and Pilot 1959). If the two are not closely related, some bridging statement and effort will have to be made. For example, in summary form, "The patient is not suicidal, but is very anxious. The following treatment is advisable."

Sometimes the question can be satisfactorily addressed by the initial assessment, with no need for continuing contact: "Patient requested referral for outpatient psychiatric treatment in her home city. Referred to Dr. X, who has agreed to see the patient on her return." In other situations, the patient is reluctant to continue or repeat the psychiatric contact, so that the advantages of ongoing monitoring and information gathering must be weighed against the disadvantages to patient, consultant, and consultee of imposing an unwanted intervention. An option that is a useful last resort is to document and discuss the patient's refusal with the medical team and then offer to carry out ongoing consultation without direct patient contact: come to the floor at intervals, read the chart, talk to involved staff members, and offer advice for diagnostic and therapeutic activities to be carried out by the primary-care team. This process, while often useful and sometimes vital, has several complications. The patient should be informed and should possibly give consent. If the patient does not consent, what should the consultant do? It may be up to the primary physician to inform the patient that he or she insists upon psychiatric advice in order to provide satisfactory care. Billing for such services is a complex matter as well. Finally, a professional always takes a risk when providing advice about a problem not viewed firsthand. Not uncommonly, the treating physician requests straightforward, finite information: What is the recommended dose of neuroleptic? Is the patient depressed? But the consultant's diagnostic process may reveal a major psychiatric illness (Golinger et al. 1985). The primary physician may not expect or request further psychiatric involvement after the question of fact is answered. However, unless the consultee actually objects, it is best to follow the patient at whatever intervals are clinically indicated, as the consultee implements the treatment plan based on the psychiatrist's observations and recommendations. The psychiatrist is best prepared to provide expert care for psychiatric conditions. A surgical consultant would not be expected to say, "Yes, the patient has acute appendicitis," and sign off a case (Rogers and Rasof 1977).

Oftentimes, even though the initial question is answered and the crisis appears to be over, it is reassuring to the primary-care team to know that the psychiatrist will remain apprised of the situation by making regular visits during the hospitalization. This is true, for example, when the patient's disordered behavior was the result of a postoperative or other delirium and has now resolved. Following patients until they are discharged from the hospital is the cautious clinical course and keeps the psychiatrist a visible participant in ongoing medical care.

On the other hand, do not hesitate to indicate to the consultee that no further psychiatric involvement is required and/or that the primary-care team can now manage the patient without assistance, on the occasions when this is clearly so. Nonpsychiatric physicians and nonphysicians sometimes believe that psychiatrists consider nearly everyone to be in need of ongoing psychiatric care. This is a good opportunity to demonstrate that a psychiatrist can give a straightforward, time-limited response to a question, or make a diagnosis of "no psychiatric disorder."

Do make sure that the original question has been answered or addressed. Immediate management problems may be so demanding that the consultant realizes only later that the primary physician had a different or related concern in mind. This concern would have been a clue to the consultee's diagnostic and therapeutic thinking about psychiatric issues. Even if it was off the mark, or perhaps especially if it was, it would have presented a teaching opportunity (Strain et al. 1985). Explain in your written and verbal communications, in a neutral and collegial fashion,

the relationship between the primary physician's observations
and your examination and conclusions.

The following case example illustrates this process:

> The psychiatrist was asked to see an elderly woman with conges-
> tive heart failure. She had been transferred from a nursing home,
> from which very little history had been transmitted, and she was
> refusing to eat. The consultation request read, "Rule out depres-
> sion." The psychiatric interview revealed that the patient was expe-
> riencing acute hallucinations and delusions. She had no signs and
> symptoms of affective disorder. She believed that the staff mem-
> bers were trying to kill her and that the hospital food was poi-
> soned. She complained that she was very hungry, but was unable
> to obtain any food that was safe to eat. It was apparent that she
> would be best treated on a psychiatric inpatient unit, and transfer
> was arranged. However, it was also important to explain,
> "Although the patient's withdrawal and inadequate food intake do
> resemble the signs of depression, they are in this case due to her
> misinterpretation of the staff's attempts to care for her."

A patient may want and/or need psychotherapy for reasons other
than those for which consultation was requested (Green 1987).
While recovering from an acute delirium following cardiac
bypass surgery, for example, the patient may realize that the
adjustment to the newly recommended life-style is going to
require a psychic confrontation with a lifelong personality style.
Many patients wish to stop smoking and appreciate a referral to
an expert in behavior modification (Abel et al. 1987). Others want
an opportunity to review their life goals and priorities with a
mental health professional. In still other cases, a medical event
triggers the recognition or exacerbation of interpersonal difficulties for which marital, family, or group treatment is indicated.

Another important issue in the consultation setting is the decision whether to initiate treatment while the patient is medically
hospitalized or to wait until the recommended outpatient psychiatric care begins. This question most commonly arises in cases of
anxiety or affective disorders that are significantly troubling to
the patient but not immediately threatening to life or long-range
health at the time of the consultation. The primary factor in favor
of the inpatient initiation of care is the ability to medically moni-

tor, by expert hospital staff, the medically ill patient's response and side effects on a 24-hour basis.

The need to initiate psychopharmacological management under medical surveillance is an acceptable medical rationale for prolonging hospitalization for a patient whose discharge has been demanded by third-party payers or utilization review bodies. If untoward complications develop, treatment can be suspended immediately and countermeasures instituted if necessary. This approach may allay the concern of the primary physician about treating a cardiac patient with tricyclic antidepressants, for example. Initiating treatment during the hospitalization also offers the patient the possibility of an expeditious therapeutic result.

Deferring treatment initiation to the outpatient psychiatrist and setting also has important advantages, especially when discharge is anticipated within days. The patient may feel different or better simply as a result of not being in the hospital, of being back in the familiar home environment, and/or of continuing to recuperate from the medical illness that occasioned the hospitalization. Or the patient may experience increased anxiety or depression in a strange new environment, or simply from being without the supportive structure and monitoring of the hospital unit.

Because it is likely that a variety of changes in medical management will have been instituted during the hospitalization, and the results, in this era of swift discharge, not fully assimilated, postponement of psychiatric treatment for some interval allows its effects to be observed and evaluated more independently of other interventions and the acute illness and recovery. Initiation of treatment in the outpatient setting allows the outpatient psychiatrist to observe the patient in the untreated condition; select, in concert with the patient and significant others, therapeutic modalities familiar to him or her; and observe and manage the response.

Repeated reference has been made to the collaboration with the primary treatment team as the cornerstone of effective consultation. The treating physician is the object of the patient's therapeutic transference and, optimally, has the patient's trust. The consultant's assessment of the patient's condition and needs is irrelevant to clinical care unless the primary physician implements the recommendations.

It is at the point of deciding upon follow-up and/or termination of the consultation that the collaboration is made manifest (Popkin and Mackenzie 1984). Either the consultant is welcomed as a member of the treatment team, so that the psychiatric recommendations are perceived and carried out as an integral part of care, or the psychiatric contact is held apart. Involvement of the primary physician in the decisions concerning follow-up and its execution cements the integration of "medical" and "psychiatric" care and facilitates the communication of this integration to the patient and family.

GOALS FOR FOLLOW-UP

The consultant can enunciate a more workable plan and better elicit the support of the consultee and patient, when the goals for follow-up are clear. Goals fall into three overlapping categories: diagnostic, therapeutic, and educational. Explicit diagnostic goals help the primary-care team accept the fact that there is insufficient evidence to arrive at a diagnostic conclusion on the basis of the initial consultation, and facilitate the observation, exploration, and documentation of the specific data necessary for the formulation of that conclusion.

For example, the elucidation of the etiology of an organic brain syndrome observed by the psychiatrist may require a variety of diagnostic tests. The staff members are more likely to order and carry out these examinations when they understand that specific treatment programs can be tailored to the diagnostic findings. On the other hand, a diagnosis of an untreatable disorder, while unfortunate, frees the staff, patient, and family from uncertainty and the need to continue to seek curative interventions. The differential diagnosis of organic brain disease may also include neurotoxic effects of treatments the patient is receiving. The psychiatrist can work with the primary team to weigh the probable risks and benefits of manipulating the dose or discontinuing the treatment in order to clarify the cause of the mental status aberration.

In many cases, diagnosis of psychiatric disorder hinges on careful observations and charting of verbalizations, vegetative signs, and behaviors of the patient. Making the goals clear is an inducement to the staff to perform and focus the required observations. The consultant may state verbally and in writing what diagnoses will be considered or ruled out by particular observations: for example, "Specific quotes from the patient will help us differentiate fear and suspicion from genuine paranoid psychosis," or, "The patient's response to benzodiazepines will be an important clue to the diagnosis of an alcohol withdrawal syndrome." Some subtleties will be detectable only directly by the psychiatrist, who will then have to explain that—and why—continued specialized psychiatric monitoring is crucial to the diagnostic process.

Therapeutic goals of follow-up require the least explanation to the consultee, because ameliorating the patient's condition is the goal of all medical care and the usual purpose of consultation. However, the nuances and specifics of therapeutic responses to psychiatric interventions are less often self-evident. Suggested treatment with medication is most familiar to primary physicians. Even though nonpsychiatrists write most of the prescriptions for psychoactive medications, expert knowledge of these agents' mechanisms of action, interactions with other drugs and conditions, and side effects is not within their areas of specialization. The consultant, again, may indicate specific signs and symptoms that are to be observed and charted by unit personnel and/or that the consultant will be monitoring.

For example, a patient's agitation may indicate either a need for a higher dose of neuroleptic or a supratherapeutic level of agents with anticholinergic side effects. The chronological relationship between the administration of the medication and the patient's agitation is an important clue to the vital discrimination between these alternatives. The consultant might recommend, "Chart patient's condition at X intervals after each neuroleptic dose," or state, "I will return at X intervals to observe the patient's response to medication." Another common situation of this kind is the withdrawal of a patient from alcohol or other substances of abuse. A suggested schedule of particular observations (for tremulousness, alertness, etc.) or of repeated visits, or an end point such as the induction of sleep, will help the primary service organize their care of the substance-abusing patient.

Primary physicians are sometimes unclear about the focused and realistic goals of treatment with psychotropic agents. For treatment with a neuroleptic, the consultant might suggest that the therapeutic aim is the control of delusions or hallucinations. With respect to an antidepressant, the issue may be the therapeutic window, or finding the optimal dose. Antidepressants are often prescribed by nonpsychiatrists in insufficient, static doses rather than gradually increased to a therapeutic level and maintained long enough to determine whether symptoms improve.

So-called "somatic" therapies other than those using psychotropic medications tend to be less familiar to nonpsychiatrists and therefore to require a different level of follow-up support. Electroconvulsive treatment, for example, can be administered to medical inpatients when they need more exacting medical monitoring than is customarily available on a psychiatric unit. "Shock treatment" is not widely well understood or accepted, and elicits considerable fear and suspicion among patients, families, and unit staff, as well as primary physicians. Follow-through with these cases often demands repeated, detailed rationales for the choice of treatment method, explanations of the method, and descriptions of the patient's probable immediate reactions and gradual recovery.

Although primary-care physicians can and do provide a wide range of effective psychosocial therapies to their patients, they do not always recognize the centrality of these interventions in the patients' improvement. Psychiatric residents, too, often underestimate the impact of their work with consultation patients on the patients' anxiety and mood. If you plan to embark on a course of psychotherapy with the patient, explain the reason for the frequency and length of the sessions. Factors include the impact of the patient's general physical condition on tolerance for extended interactions, the opportunity to accomplish a piece of definitive or facilitating work while the patient is in the hospital, the need for intensive support during a medical and/or psychosocial crisis, the need to monitor response, and the patient's estimated capacity for insight (Blacher 1984). The psychiatric consultant can indicate, "We will assess the need for anxiolytics after we have observed the effect of daily, brief, supportive psychotherapy sessions on the patient's condition," or, "The patient may be greatly cheered by an explanation of her optimistic prognosis." Follow-up work may also include helping the patient's family, religious institution, or a social welfare service assist the patient.

Each of the foregoing follow-up goals is educational as well as diagnostic and/or therapeutic. Some aspects of the educational process are immediately useful to the patient. Teaching the staff about the individual patient's dynamics and how to deal in general with patients with various personality structures enables care providers to work more empathically and effectively (Reichard 1964). Helping the patient to note connections between life events, feelings, medical illnesses, relationships with medical personnel, and medical interventions is a goal simultaneously educational and therapeutic. Follow-up can also include explicitly educational activities. Whether the consultant returns to the unit with relevant articles from the psychiatric literature, elucidates the workings of the process of crisis intervention, or describes the usual psychological concomitants of a given medical/surgical condition or procedure, the consultee service comes away with a greater knowledge base to apply to ensuing clinical and educational situations. We have never found that the consultant becomes superfluous. There are always new students and staff to educate, and those with whom one has worked over time make more sophisticated use of consultation services.

IMPLEMENTATION

As indicated above, once need is demonstrated and goals are enunciated, the consultant must outline clear and detailed plans for the nature and timing of follow-up activities. Note in the chart exactly what follow-up is planned and who is expected to participate. Are you going to call or write to family members, nursing home or school personnel, or previous therapists? When? How will the data obtained affect your recommendations? Indicate that the patient has given consent. Sometimes the patient refuses to allow the consultant to inform others about his condition, but will compromise by allowing the consultant to contact others only to gather information, providing this data is shared with the patient. Sometimes the patient will agree that you interview a friend or relative only in his or her presence, or on the telephone with the patient on an extension receiver.

Perhaps you plan to meet with family members or others. Make a prominent note in the chart, as early as possible, indicating the time and place of the meeting. Make it clear whether the participation of staff members is not anticipated, or whether they are highly encouraged to attend, and if so, what information they should bring, what roles they might play, and to what ends. Ask that they let you know in advance so that you can secure an appropriate space for the number of participants, plan the meeting, and inform the family. Indicate also how you are going to consult with, supervise, or collaborate with other staff members, such as social workers, psychologists, and occupational therapists.

Carry out, and reassess at appropriate intervals, the precise diagnostic observations required. Does the patient's response to environmental manipulations and interpersonal events point to a situational reaction rather than a major affective disorder? When the laboratory values whose need you elaborated in your first note are entered in the chart, indicate that you have noted them, how they correlate with the patient's clinical condition, and how they affect the differential diagnosis and treatment plan. For example, the fact that the toxicology screen revealed hallucinogens, and that the patient's psychotic symptoms are decreasing, diminishes the likelihood that a patient's psychotic symptoms were due only to schizophrenia (Svarstad 1979). The fact that the patient claims to be unable to walk but has been observed smoking cigarettes that were left well out of reach reinforces a hypothesis of malingering.

Of particular concern is evidence of the assimilation and application of the psychiatric consultation in the ensuing notes and behavior of the primary-service team. Have they ordered the tests, other consultations, changes in management, or psychotropic agents recommended (Moses and Barzilay 1967)? Have the observations you advised been made and entered into the chart? Is there evidence of a change in staff's attitudes toward the patient? For example, have they offered more explanations of illness processes, procedures, and treatments? Do their progress notes reflect increased understanding of the patient's attitudes and behaviors? For example, a patient who was regarded as "paranoid" may have been found by the consultant to be of borderline normal intelligence, uninformed, and frightened. After these findings have been explicated, staff notes will refer to the state of the patient's "anxiety" rather than to his or her lack of cooperation (Svarstad 1979). Consultees who have integrated psychiatric formulations will also tend to ask new, relevant questions and offer new, relevant data.

If your recommendations have not been implemented, why

not? The psychiatric consultant treads a careful path, utilizing psychosocial and psychodynamic skills to try to understand the thinking, feeling, and resistances of consultees in the interests of education and patient care, without "psychoanalyzing" consultees in a clinical or patronizing manner. You may realize that the primary physician cannot tolerate, or is overly susceptible to, certain of the patient's character traits; for example, he or she is put off by a patient who vies for control of the medical treatment, or is overwhelmed by a dependent and clinging patient. Perhaps it will become apparent that the real agenda was to dispose of the patient's case in some way or that there is interpersonal conflict among members of the staff that is being played out in the arena of your suggestions. Possibly you did not make the rationale for the interventions fully clear to the relevant care providers or did not realize budgetary, time, or other constraints under which the care providers work. Further interventions must be focused on your assessment of their failure to follow up.

Another aspect of the implementation phase of the consultation is the assessment of the results of the psychiatric interventions themselves, and the ongoing adjustment of psychiatric treatment. Psychotropic medications and dosages will have to be titrated to therapeutic response and side effects. Note whether recommended medical interventions had the desired effects: Did the administration of oxygen to the hypoxic patient improve his or her mental status?

Assimilate the results of psychosocial interventions into the ongoing differential diagnosis and treatment plan. Did the introduction of a clock and calendar facilitate the orientation of the patient suffering from an organic brain syndrome? If so, other orienting devices, such as charts, newspapers, etc., may also be helpful. If not, future plans may need to be predicated on the patient's chronic disorientation. Was the patient's agitation allayed by the presence of a family member or "sitter" during the night? If so, facilitate the relative's or sitter's continued availability. If not, investigate whether there is something in this particular relationship that is not helpful to the patient, or whether some other management is required. Has the provision for child care at home, or arrangement for safekeeping of the Social Security check, enabled the patient to better tolerate a medically optimal length of stay in the hospital?

The follow-up period, no matter how brief, is an excellent opportunity to assess the patient's psychological response to psychiatric contact. Many patients feel better immediately after reviewing the course of their medical and psychological problems, ventilating their feelings, and having the experience of being listened to and understood by a psychiatrist. They begin to ponder the relationships between life events and conflicts and episodes of symptom onset or exacerbation—that is, to acquire insight. It also becomes clear whether or not the patient is likely to be interested in, follow through with, and benefit from additional psychotherapy.

If the patient is medically and psychologically able, and the hospitalization is longer than a day or two, brief psychotherapy, or crisis intervention, can be accomplished in the medical setting (Bellak and Small 1965). Although consultation patients are not generally self-referred, do not see themselves as "psychiatric" patients, and are preoccupied with their medical illnesses and treatments, those who are psychologically symptomatic can be highly motivated to engage in the psychotherapeutic process. Concentration on their inner dynamics can be a welcome relief and distraction from lying in a hospital bed waiting for the next venipuncture. The stress of illness and treatment heightens their need for human contact, interest, and understanding. The psychiatrist, being medically trained, is in an excellent position to comprehend the clinical situation in its entirety.

Discharge Planning

Not uncommonly, some sort of discharge planning is the motivation for the consultation. The primary-care team wishes that the consultant would "take" the difficult-to-manage patient, is not sure whether the patient can manage independent living after hospitalization, or is concerned whether a patient who wishes to leave without completing medically indicated workup or treatment is competent to make that decision. In every case, the consultant must determine whether outpatient or inpatient psychiatric care is indicated, and how to facilitate compliance if it is.

In general discharge planning, the psychiatric consultant is a specialized member of the medical team. Unless transfer to an inpatient psychiatric unit is contemplated, responsibility for discharge planning does not center on the consultant, although other team members may wish, or even insist, this were so. The fact that the patient has psychiatric problems does not automatically make him or her the primary patient of the consultant. Appropriate consultation functions include expert mental status examinations, with special emphasis on the patient's ability to apply cognitive skills to the necessities of daily life outside the hospital: "How do you prepare your dinner?" "Describe how you get to the doctor's office from your house." "If you buy a loaf of bread for $1.59, how much change will you get from a $5 bill?"

The interpretation of proverbs is a less useful parameter than the ability to describe the steps in obtaining food and cooking a meal, and the ability to make change in the grocery store is more important than the accuracy of serial seven subtraction. Psychoses, affective disorders, and anxiety disorders may not be severe enough to demand inpatient treatment, but they may still be a central factor in decisions about the patient's optimal placement after discharge. Where will the patient be most free from added stress, feel most useful and self-sufficient, be most likely to follow the necessary medical regimen, and seek additional help if deteriorating?

Assessments of need and motivation for outpatient psychiatric care must be integrated with the practical realities of care available. Patients are most likely to see an outpatient psychiatrist when he or she is the consultant seen in the hospital. Simply meeting a new therapist before discharge, or visiting the outpatient facility on a pass, increases the likelihood of continued treatment. What sort of care can the patient afford or finance with the help of private or government insurance coverage? What are the mental health resources of the community in which the patient lives? Can the patient obtain transportation? In terms of clear thinking, education, and charting for medicolegal purposes, it is important to distinguish one kind of treatment limitation from another. The note in the chart should reflect clear, feasible, rationally supported plans, and not musings on the inadequacy of the mental health and/or insurance system.

ENDING THE CONSULTATION

A psychiatric consultation may end, by plan or default, any time between the moment the request for consultation is made and the discharge of the patient. While a consultant may continue to see the patient, in collaboration with the primary-care team, after the patient leaves the hospital, such contact no longer constitutes consultation as construed in this manual. Some consultations are designated "brief" or "limited" from the beginning. The consultant seeks a limited kind of information: a medication dosage, the name of a referral facility, etc. If the consultant agrees that the clinical situation does not demand further involvement, the consultation ends after the desired information is conveyed. Telephone or face-to-face communication allows the consultee to confirm that the consultation has been satisfactory. The written consultation includes a statement that no further contact is desired or necessary, often with an invitation to call the consultant again if the need arises.

Many consultation contacts continue through the medical hospitalization. Hospitalizations tend to be very short, and there is little enough time to complete a full assessment, make a diagnosis, recommend treatment, and adjust it to the clinical response of the patient. Prolonged hospitalizations are usually limited to complex and serious conditions and treatments. These are enormously stressful to patients. This stress can be alleviated by ongoing psychiatric care (Levitan and Kornfeld 1981). So that there will be no misunderstanding or anxiety, the consultant can write "will follow" in the note following each session. It does happen that the need for and/or possibility of psychiatric follow-up end during the hospitalization. This is not uncommon in patients who have an acute organic brain syndrome during a fulminant infection, metabolic imbalance, or postoperative period. After cognitive recovery, and a period in which the psychiatrist and primary-care team help the patient understand and accept the episode of disordered thinking and behavior, the patient may be quite able to convalesce without further psychiatric intervention.

A consultation occasioned by a misunderstanding or miscommunication between the staff, patient, and/or significant others, which can be corrected in a visit or two, can also be ended before the patient is discharged. There are advantages to ending selected consultations before discharge. The ability to identify an end to the need for psychiatric care reinforces the concepts that some psychiatric illnesses are finite and many people do not require psychiatric attention. It is reassuring to the patient to be told that there is no further need for psychiatric care.

A very small number of patients adamantly refuse to see the consultant again; after attempts to understand and address the patient's stance, and in the absence of an acute problem interfering with the patient's health or care, the psychiatrist may agree to withdraw. Occasionally a relative may demand an end to follow-up. Remember that, until or unless adjudicated incompetent, the adult patient alone has the right to make decisions about his or her care.

At whatever point in the patient's hospitalization the consultation ends, as throughout the process of consultation, make sure the consultee is informed and preferably in agreement. While we do not want to foster the impression that psychiatric intervention, once solicited, is self-perpetuating and endless, we are equally invested in preventing situations in which the primary service feels abandoned—and situations in which the consultant is pressured into an inappropriate primary-care role. Once all are in agreement, chart a brief summary of the reasons the consultation was requested, the process and outcome of the consultation, and the reasoning behind its conclusion. The consultee will have a succinct representation of the clinical situation and the reasons for the recommended course of action, will be more likely to facilitate the patient's cooperation, and will perceive the psychiatric consultation as a focused and clinically pertinent process.

REFERENCES

Abel GG, Rouleau J-L, Coyne BJ: Behavioral medicine strategies in medical patients, in Principles of Medical Psychiatry. Edited by Stoudemire MD, Fogel BS. Orlando, FL, Grune & Stratton, 1987, pp 329–345

Bellak L, Small L: Emergency Psychotherapy and Brief Psychotherapy. New York, Grune & Stratton, 1965

Blacher RS: The briefest encounter: psychotherapy for medical and surgical patients. Gen Hosp Psychiatry 6:226–232, 1984

Garrick TR, Stotland NL: How to write a psychiatric consultation. Am J Psychiatry 139:849–855, 1982

Golinger R, Teitelbaum ML, Folstein MF: Clarity of request for consultation: its relationship to psychiatric diagnosis. Psychosomatics 26:649–653, 1985

Green SA: Principles of medical psychotherapy, in Principles of Medical Psychiatry. Edited by Stoudemire MD, Fogel BS. Orlando, FL, Grune & Stratton, 1987, pp 1–21

Karasu TB, Plutchnik R, Conte H, et al: What do physicians want from a psychiatric consultation service? Compr Psychiatry 18:73–81, 1977

Levitan SJ, Kornfeld DS: Clinical and cost benefits of liaison psychiatry. Am J Psychiatry 138:790–793, 1981

Lipowski ZJ: Consultation-liaison psychiatry: an overview. Am J Psychiatry 131:623–630, 1974

Moses R, Barzilay S: The influence of psychiatric consultation on the course of illness in the general hospital patient. Compr Psychiatry 8:16–26, 1967

Popkin MK, Mackenzie TB: Communicating with the referring physician, in Manual of Psychiatric Consultation and Emergency Care. Edited by Guggenheim FG, Weiner MF. New York, Jason Aronson, 1984, pp 115–123

Reichard JF: Teaching principles of medical psychology to medical house officers: methods and problems, in Psychiatry and Medical Practice in a General Hospital. Edited by Zinberg NE. New York, International Universities Press, 1964, pp 169–204

Rogers RR, Rasof B: The gap between psychiatric practice and the medical model. Compr Psychiatry 18:459–463, 1977

Schiff SK, Pilot ML: An approach to psychiatric care in the general hospital. Arch Gen Psychiatry 1:349–357, 1959

Strain JJ, Pincus HA, Houpt JL, et al: Models of mental health training for primary care physicians. Psychosom Med 47:95–109, 1985

Svarstad BL: Physician-patient communication and patient conformity with medical advice, in Health, Illness, and Medicine: A Reader in Medical Sociology. Edited by Albrecht GL, Higgins PC. Chicago, IL, Rand McNally, 1979, pp 243–259

11

Role of the Consultation-Liaison Psychiatrist as a Medical Educator

This chapter outlines the various teaching settings in which the consultation-liaison psychiatrist operates. As the "liaison" in consultation-liaison suggests, the psychiatrist does more than provide patient-specific, physician-requested consultations. In addition, the psychiatrist works to become an integral member of the medical/surgical team and to educate nonpsychiatrists about psychiatrically relevant aspects of patient care (Lipowski 1974). First, the chapter will explore the role that the consultation-liaison psychiatrist plays in training nonpsychiatric physicians, particularly while those physicians are training as residents. Second, this outline suggests why the consultation-liaison psychiatrist is ideally suited to actively teach psychiatric residents; the consultation-liaison psychiatrist can act both as a role model for the psychiatrist-physician and as a specialist in syndromes on the border between psychiatric and somatic, such as irritable bowel syndrome, conversion, and hypochondriasis. Finally, as an active member of the medical-school teaching faculty, the consultation-liaison psychiatrist can show medical students how a patient's psychiatric status affects all medical diagnosis and treatment.

TRAINING OF NONPSYCHIATRIC PHYSICIANS

In the general hospital, consultation-liaison psychiatrists educate other medical specialists about how to identify, assess, refer, and, on occasion, manage their patients. This process of education is important because most patients with mental illness present to medical settings where few of them are appropriately recognized and referred for proper treatment (Regier et al. 1978). How much psychiatric management can or should nonpsychiatric medical practitioners actually handle, and to what extent should psychiatrists "collude" in this? Although these patients fall within the bounds of psychiatry, nonpsychiatric physicians are the primary "consumers" of our "product" (consultations and liaison activities), and our educational work must aim, in part, to foster future referrals (Wise 1987). The consultation-liaison psychiatrist should educate the nonpsychiatric client in potential risks and dangers associated with psychiatric management.

For example, although psychotherapy is an important component of the management of psychiatric illness, nonpsychiatric physicians are rarely trained in this therapy and cannot be quickly taught it. Obviously, nonpsychiatric physicians cannot be taught how to manage psychiatric illness in a few consultations or a single lecture; to argue differently would undermine the image and reality that psychiatry is a specialty like other medical specialties. Certainly, no psychiatrist would presume to manage thyroiditis after obtaining an endocrine consult or perform a colectomy for ulcerative colitis after attending a surgery lecture. Today, most major illnesses are treated by specialists.

Keeping current in these medical areas helps the consultant recognize the psychiatric components of these diseases. Similarly, nonpsychiatric medical practitioners need to learn how to obtain emotional and cognitive information about their patients, to have a high index of suspicion to appreciate the high prevalence of psychiatric disorders possibly effecting the presentation of medical illness, to recognize psychiatric illness, to make informed working diagnoses using rigorous criteria, and to understand what psychiatric care entails. Primary-care physicians often need to be guided and encouraged to talk directly with their patients about their emotional state, and their reactions to illness and loss, in order to provide medical treatment most effectively (Iwasaki 1979). If the primary-care physician is taught to recognize a patient's usual coping styles, then he or she can better manage reactions to illness and recommend treatments or hospitalization (Geringer and Stern 1986).

Psychiatrists may also fear that nonpsychiatric physicians will be encouraged to use psychopharmacological agents, when they already prescribe many more of them than do psychiatrists (Balter 1973). Because they are untrained in psychotherapy, nonpsychiatric physicians tend to see psychopharmacology as the only psychiatric modality. The nonpsychiatric physician who depends on pharmacological agents may not recognize the importance of thorough psychiatric evaluation and treatment.

The psychiatric profession is currently examining the extent to which primary-care physicians are taught certain aspects of psychiatric diagnosis and treatment. As reviewed by Burns et al. (1983), primary-care professional organizations such as the American Board of Internal Medicine, the American Academy of Pediatrics, and the American Medical Association have recommended educating primary caregivers in using the physician-patient relationship as a therapeutic tool, in becoming aware of and understanding the behavioral and psychosocial aspects of illness, and in recognizing and managing psychiatric disorders and emotional problems. Strain et al. (1985) suggest that in the future, primary-care physicians should be trained in psychosomatic medicine, psychophysiological reactions, and the interactions between biologic, psychologic, and social factors in health and disease. Primary-care physicians should be familiar with these areas and have some expertise in diagnosis and referral, particularly because between 15% and 50% of all patients visiting primary-care physicians have some emotional or cognitive disorder (Hoeper et al. 1979). This educational focus of psychiatric consultation is suited to every level in medical training. And because the consultation-liaison process opens up the usually private psychiatrist-patient encounter, the process is well suited to training purposes.

Throughout this manual we have discussed opportunities to teach nonpsychiatric physicians about the psychiatric issues specific to their patients. This education can involve learning how to interpret patient behavior, how to mediate between the patient and staff, and how to make specific recommendations for management. According to Strain et al. (1985), primary-care physicians can be taught mental health–related concepts and skills through six program types: consultation, liaison, bridge, hybrid, autonomous, and postgraduate specialization. In the consultation model, the psychiatric-consultation team teaches through specific patient consults. The team focuses only minimally on psychiatric diagnosis and treatment skills. Instead, the team works to increase the consulting service's awareness of psychiatric morbidity, guiding basic psychopharmacology and effective referral. These services are provided by the psychiatric department. The liaison model is similar, but it also provides for attendance by psychiatrists at patient-care conferences, rounds, and/or participation in medical-service rounds. The bridge model involves more extensive, formal teaching of psychiatric methods and encourages the primary-care faculty to involve themselves in teaching. This model also emphasizes teaching interviewing and treatment skills. The psychiatric service provides a longitudinal presence on the medical service that allows the psychiatrist to develop a stronger relationship with members of the service and to more accurately identify their educational needs. The hybrid model expands the bridge model to integrate psychosocial education into every aspect of primary-care education experience with diverse and direct involvement by other mental health professionals such as social workers and psychologists. The autonomous model involves fully integrated teaching in mental health managed by the primary-care specialty without significant involvement from members of the psychiatry department. The postgraduate specialization model involves the primary-care physician functioning on rotations in psychiatric specialties as the mental health specialist. The optimal model is viewed as specific to local needs and goals.

TRAINING PSYCHIATRIC RESIDENTS IN CONSULTATION-LIAISON

Consultation-liaison psychiatry provides psychiatrists with the opportunity to renew and enrich medical knowledge and contacts. General psychiatry residents are expected to spend at least one-third of a year on consultation-liaison psychiatry (Accreditation Council 1987). The formal objectives of such rotations have been presented in detail elsewhere (Cohen-Cole et al. 1982; Mohl and Cohen-Cole 1985). The Association for Academic Psychiatry appointed a task force to formulate objectives for residency training. Tables 11-1 and 11-2 summarize and condense the topics considered essential by this task force. (For details, see Cohen-Cole et al.'s [1982] lucid work.) The task force objectives include recommendations for what information the trainee should learn as well as what skills he or she should develop.

The resident is expected to develop a comprehensive understanding of the consultation process, including specific roles and responsibilities of the consultant in the medical setting. For example, the resident should learn the biopsychosocial dimensions of medical practice and medical disorders, including the effects of psychological and social variables in the onset, course, and outcome. The resident should also be educated about specific psychiatric syndromes such as delirium, somatoform disorders, and sexual dysfunction in medical patients; behavioral disorders resulting from medications and anxiety; and dysfunctional behaviors such as obesity. The resident is expected to develop a broad understanding of the principles behind the various treatment modalities used in consultation-liaison settings, including psychopharmacology, electroconvulsive treatment, crisis intervention, behavior therapy in medical patients, and the possible role of nonmedical therapists in providing certain aspects of treatment. Finally, the psychiatric resident is expected to develop a variety of skills: gathering data from the patient, medical charts, and consulting physician; formulating cases along several dimensions (including biological, social, psychological, and legal dimensions); and providing an organized, well-reasoned treatment strategy, which might include other therapists, environmental manipulations in the medical center, etc.

The need for medical knowledge in the consultation-liaison rotation is often difficult for the psychiatrist in training. Insecurities related to rusty diagnostic and treatment skills often surface. The psychiatric resident may find it especially difficult to relate as a senior house officer to house officers in other specialties. Psychiatric residents may find themselves caught between an insecure identity as a psychiatrist and a rapidly fading identity as a medical doctor. They may be curt or hostile with consulting physicians, in the preconscious hope of foreshortening a contact that they feel may reveal their anxiety. Alternatively, they may behave

Table 11-1. Knowledge objectives for residents in consultation-liaison psychiatry

A. Consultation process

    1. Consultant: objectives, responsibilities, authority, and limitations of psychiatric consultation in medical settings

    2. Consultation relationship: consultation vs. supervision, referrals, or psychotherapy

    3. Factors influencing the initiation, process, and outcome of consultation

    4. Types of consultations: patient-, physician-, program-, and nurse-centered

B. Biopsychosocial dimensions of medical practice

    1. Influence of psychological and social variables on predisposition, onset, course, and outcome of somatic illness

    2. Psychological/social adaptation to illness

    3. Caregiver's reactions to patients

    4. General systems theory approaches to understanding the dynamics of illness and recuperation

C. Clinical syndromes

    1. Psychiatric conditions

        a. Delirium/dementia and organic brain syndrome

        b. Somatoform disorders

        c. Factitious disorders

        d. Depression in medical conditions

        e. Drug and alcohol dependence, intoxication, and/or withdrawal

        f. Psychological factors affecting physical conditions

        g. Sexual dysfunction in medical patients

    2. Behavioral conditions

        a. Behavioral side effects of medications

        b. Nonadherence to medical and treatment regimens

        c. Grief, death, and dying

        d. Anxiety in the medical setting

        e. Personality problems affecting medical care in the hospital

        f. Suicidal/homicidal threats in medical patients

        g. Obesity

        h. Sleep disorders in medical patients

        i. Chronic pain

D. Treatments[a]

    1. Organic psychiatric treatments for medical patients

   a. Psychotropic medication treatment for conditions listed above under "Clinical syndromes," including antianxiety, antidepressant, and antipsychotic medications, and lithium
   b. Effects of various illnesses on prescribing practices for psychotropic medication
   c. Electroconvulsive therapy in medical patients

2. Nonorganic treatments

   a. Crisis intervention
   b. Individual brief psychotherapy
   c. Family therapy
   d. Behavior therapy, including cognitive-behavior therapy, skills training, biofeedback, contingency management, token economy, systematic exposure, and behavioral analysis
   f. Intervention by nonpsychiatric medical personnel such as physical therapists, diabetes nurse specialists, psychologists, social workers, nurses, etc.
   g. Other treatments such as hypnosis, relaxation training, etc.
   h. Patient education

---

[a]While residents are not expected to be versatile in all treatments listed, an understanding of indications, contraindications, and appropriate referral is essential.
Source. Abstracted from Cohen-Cole et al. 1982.

as if they know less than they actually do. The "I'm just a shrink" retort is analogous to the "I'm just a surgeon" retort by the surgeon confronted with complex psychosocial problems. Most often, the resident simply suppresses those moments of ignorance.

These patterns and others impede the learning process and may actually detract from good clinical care by covering over the resident's gaps in knowledge about the patient. As discussed in Chapter 9, psychiatric residents must be taught to recognize their limitations and encouraged to tell primary physicians, "I don't know," when they reach those limits. The primary physician is in a similar position: he or she too may not fully understand the patient and his or her problems. When both clinicians identify the lacunae in their understanding of the patient, they can work together to help each other fill in the gaps.

The working relationship the resident establishes with a senior psychiatric consultant may provide a useful model for a mature physician-psychiatrist relationship with a nonpsychiatric physician. In turn, those mature relationships facilitate the interdisciplinary clinical work that allows physicians to assimilate vast

Table 11-2. Skills objectives for residents in consultation-liaison psychiatry

A. Data gathering

  1. Obtain history from patient, medical chart, and/or referring physician, and from relevant other sources.

B. Case formulation

  1. Biological, psychological, and social contributions
  2. Nonverbalized agenda of consultee in consultations
  3. Biological, psychological, and social interventions appropriate to particular consultation
  4. Elements of a consultation report
  5. Legal issues impinging upon case management

C. Intervention

  1. Organization and teaching of nonpsychiatric personnel
  2. Choosing treatment strategies appropriate to the medical setting
  3. Use of behavioral management techniques appropriate to the medical setting
  4. Recognition and utilization of emotional reactions that arise among ward staff, referring physician, and psychiatric consultant
  5. Management of nonadherence in medical settings

Source. Abstracted, with minor revisions, from Cohen-Cole et al. 1982.

increases in medical knowledge and treatment and use that new knowledge to treat and solve clinical problems. As part of this complex web of interacting generalists and specialists, the psychiatric consultant acts as an arbiter. The resident on the consultation service works with residents and attending physicians in other disciplines and through that working relationship can acquire updated medical knowledge and establish long-term relationships with peers in other specialties. Gaining clinical experience and being observed by senior physicians in this role help the psychiatric resident in the sea of medical specialists and nonmedical psychological counselors secure a self-image as a psychiatrist.

The consultation service is often one of the few services in a training program where the resident actually evaluates and treats patients in the presence of senior members of the faculty. Apprenticeship is one of the best modes of learning. The consultation service provides an opportunity for the senior clinician to directly observe how the resident and patient interact, to provide immediate feedback to the resident, and, on occasion, to suggest alternatives to the resident during on-the-spot therapeutic interaction. The following case example illustrates the efficacy of this approach:

> A psychiatric resident began performing an interview on an elderly patient in obvious pain from a gangrenous leg. The resident immediately began exploring the presumed depression for which the psychiatrists were consulted. The patient was uninterested in answering the resident's questions and asked to have the interview terminated, despite the resident's repeated efforts to obtain information about the patient's mood. The struggling resident looked for help to the attending physician, who began asking the patient about his obvious physical pain. The patient, who had not received a pain medication in several hours, explained that the pain was very discouraging and that it was difficult to get pain medication when it was needed because the nurses were very busy. At that point, the attending physician and resident contacted a nurse to provide pain medication. The patient was both grateful and able to provide the necessary history without delay.

Through such observations, the faculty are also able to accurately evaluate the resident's interviewing, diagnostic, and treatment skills. During the consultation-liaison service rotation, the psychiatric resident learns to develop and communicate rapid, clear diagnostic and treatment formulations.

Consultation-liaison psychiatry also offers concentrated exposure to clinical case examples that are infrequently found in other clinical settings. For example, consultation-liaison psychiatry exposes the resident to organic brain syndromes, the psychiatric effects of medical drugs, acute reactions to catastrophic medical illness and loss, and the psychiatric concomitants of medical conditions. Although rarely presenting in psychiatric clinics, patients with clinical conditions such as Munchausen syndrome and other factitious illnesses, Briquet's syndrome, and other forms of somatization disorder are relatively common on medical wards. In fact, the consultation situation offers the complete range of psychological conditions affecting physical disorder and conversion disorder, and other psychiatric conditions where the patient is loath to undergo psychiatric treatment (such as schizoid and antisocial personality disorders).

The teaching service is typically structured around several didactic activities. An introductory lecture series covers the critical topics in psychosomatic medicine and consultation-liaison psychiatry (Tables 11-1 and 11-2). Important literature in the field (Mohl and Cohen-Cole 1985) is often best covered in this format. A formal case conference in which the psychiatric resident presents the details of the patient history and hospital course followed by an interview and discussion by senior consultation-liaison or guest interviewers provides an opportunity for trainees to observe differing approaches to clinical problem solving. The strength of any clinical service is in the supervised, in-depth intake, workup, and treatment of a wide variety of patients. Early in a resident's consultation-liaison experience, we recommend that the staff psychiatrist be present for all phases of workup. Later, the more traditional format of patient presentation by the resident followed by patient interview (as needed) by the senior supervising clinician can be used. While there are no set rules on the frequency of rounds, optimal learning is fostered in an environment where the resident is allowed a wide range of autonomy, with a supervisor readily available.

We consider it inappropriate for consultation-liaison services to be provided by residents who have primary responsibility for other major clinical services, such as an inpatient ward. Similarly, we consider it a suboptimal situation for supervising physicians to be primarily involved in nonconsultation-liaison activities. We believe that medical/surgical wards deserve strong, specialized psychiatric support because there is such a high rate of psychiatric disorders in medical inpatients, such a great number of psychiatric conditions mimicking medical disease, and such a great number of psychiatric complications resulting from medical illness and treatments.

TRAINING OF MEDICAL STUDENTS IN CONSULTATION-LIAISON PSYCHIATRY

Medical students also find consultation-liaison psychiatry to be an ideal training experience. Consultation-liaison psychiatry is perceived as relevant to training in all clinical areas. The student experiences the mechanics of the physician-psychiatrist interacting with other medical and surgical specialists in clinical situations that display the roles of both. Consultation work confronts the medical student with the impossibility of the mind-body dichotomy. The student learns to recognize that psychological conditions affecting medical disorders reveal how a patient's emotional state dramatically alters the presentation of medical illness. Through encounters with somatization and factitious disorders, the student is challenged to differentiate "somatic" from apparently "somatic" conditions. When psychological reactions to medical illness and death arouse normal compassion, those reactions expose the student to the natural process of mourning. Finally, consultation-liaison exposes the student to an important concomitant of "differential diagnosis," namely, how several levels of psychological and biological factors are integrated into a disease process. Those students who are not primarily interested in psychiatry recognize that they will confront problems in their future careers requiring referral to or consultation with a psychiatrist.

Medical-student training also significantly shapes a physician's basic attitudes toward patient care (Schuffel 1979). During medical school, students learn the important coping strategies for dealing with difficult or complicated patient situations (such as death, character pathology, or family disruption); these strategies become the prototypes of strategies they will depend on throughout their career. Thus, the psychiatric consultant plays a key role in helping the student identify and work through the problematic affects associated with difficult patient situations.

REFERENCES

Accreditation Council for Graduate Medical Education: Special requirements for residency training in psychiatry, in 1987–1988 Directory of Graduate Medical Education Programs. Chicago, IL, American Medical Association, 1987, Sect 21, pp 85–90

Balter MB: An analysis of psychotherapeutic drug consumption in the United States, in Proceedings of the Anglo-American Conference on Drug Abuse: Etiology of Drug Abuse, Vol 1. Edited by Bowen RA. London, Royal Society of Medicine, 1973, pp 58–65

Burns B, Scott J, Burke J, et al: Mental health training of primary care residents: a review of recent literature (1974–1981). Gen Hosp Psychiatry 5:157–169, 1983

Cohen-Cole SA, Haggerty J, Raft D: Objectives for residents in consultation psychiatry: recommendations of a task force. Psychosomatics 23:703–708, 1982

Geringer ES, Stern TA: Coping with medical illness: the impact of personality types. Psychosomatics 27:251–261, 1986

Hoeper EU, et al: Estimated prevalence of RDC mental disorder in primary medical care. Int J Ment Health 8:6–15, 1979

Iwasaki T: Teaching liaison psychiatry and clinical practice of psychosomatic medicine in the general hospital, in The Teaching of Psychosomatic Medicine and Consultation-Liaison Psychiatry. Edited by Kimball CP, Krakowski AJ. Bibliotheca Psychiatrica No 159. Basel, S Karger, 1979, pp 32–38

Lipowski ZJ: Consultation-liaison psychiatry: an overview. Am J Psychiatry 131:623–630, 1974

Mohl PC, Cohen-Cole SA: Basic readings in consultation psychiatry. Psychosomatics 26:, 1985

Regier DA, Goldberg ID, Taube CA: De facto U.S. mental health services system. Arch Gen Psychiatry 35:685–693, 1978

Schuffel W: Training in anger: how not to communicate with one's medical seniors, in The Teaching of Psychosomatic Medicine and Consultation-Liaison Psychiatry. Edited by Kimball CP, Krakowski AJ. Bibliotheca Psychiatrica No 159, Basel, S Karger, 1979, pp 32–38

Strain JJ, Pincus HA, Houpt JL, et al: Models of mental health training for primary care physicians. Psychosom Med 47:95–110, 1985

Wise TN: Segmenting and accessing the market in consultation-liaison psychiatry. Gen Hosp Psychiatry 9:354–359, 1987

12

Consultation-Liaison in a Changing World of Psychiatry

Today, medical care is rapidly evolving: costs are skyrocketing, funding is shrinking, information is expanding, and technology is advancing at an unprecedented pace. In this changing world psychiatrists cannot afford to ignore these exigencies, because they have the potential to both hurt and foster the practice of consultation-liaison psychiatry.

Now, as always, determinants change so rapidly that it is too difficult to predict the future. However, by shrinking the focus of the practitioner, medical subspecialization has led to an increase in the involvement of consultation-liaison psychiatrists in medical and surgical services. Unlike other specialists, the consultation-liaison psychiatrist is knowledgeable about both the emotional and the physical aspects of illness. That double knowledge is important, because between 1973 and 1982, for example, the number of patients discharged with a primary diagnosis of mental disorder more than doubled (Larson et al. 1987). In general hospitals without psychiatric units, between 1965 and 1979, the number of patients discharged with mental disorder diagnoses increased six-fold. As these statistics suggest, many patients on medical wards need psychiatric treatment, and the consultation-liaison psychiatrist—when available—has become the specialist of choice (Larson et al. 1987). Indeed, about 25% of all psychiatrists today engage in some consultation and/or liaison practice (Larson et al. 1987).

205

In the preceding chapters, we have analyzed the process of consultation-liaison psychiatry. And now we will outline how the newer realities of the medical-care system will be integrated into the practice of consultation-liaison psychiatry. First, we will review how consultation-liaison psychiatry benefits the medical unit. Then, we will examine how reimbursement issues have affected the funding of consultation-liaison psychiatry and how consultation-liaison psychiatry cuts the cost of health care in the long run. Finally, we will discuss the psychiatric consultant's responsibility for helping inpatient wards cope with stress, for quality assurance standards, and for keeping up with a range of medicolegal issues.

THE BENEFITS OF CONSULTATION-LIAISON PSYCHIATRY TO THE MEDICAL UNIT

Diagnosis

Consultation-liaison psychiatrists specialize in a broad range of diagnosis essential to caring for patients on medical and surgical wards, including somatization, psychological conditions that affect physical disorders, factitious disorders, psychiatric complications of medical or street drugs and medical conditions, differential diagnosis of acute and chronic organic brain dysfunction, and sexual disorders of medical patients. Although oriented to psychiatric complications, the consultation-liaison psychiatrist's diagnostic skill depends on how well he or she evaluates medical symptoms. Medical and surgical practitioners commonly refer patients for psychiatric evaluation because they wonder whether the apparent symptoms of somatic disease are "real." Trained in medical and psychiatric diagnosis, the consultant can review the medical workup to determine whether it is complete and whether it treats the symptom consistently, and then integrate the workup with the data from the psychiatric assessment in order to arrive at a differential diagnosis.

By contrast, nonpsychiatric physicians often impute certain symptoms to anxiety or depression and thus prematurely question the significance of other symptoms and signs. For example, ulcerative colitis can cause abdominal cramping without melena triggered by minor daily stresses. Frustrated with an unpredictably, yet consistently relapsing disease, the physicians may prefer to attribute all of the new symptomatology to "stress" and feel as if they are doing their patients a favor when they send them to the psychiatrist. Similarly, the medical diagnostician may be so distracted by psychotic fantasies of delirious patients that he or she is unable to diagnose frank brain dysfunction. In such cases, the medical practitioner clearly lacks the training that allows the consultation-liaison psychiatrist to integrate psychiatric and medical assessments into a balanced diagnosis.

As discussed in Chapter 9, the consultation-liaison psychiatrist must work closely with the primary medical team to determine which medical tests are important for differential diagnosis. Thus, for example, certain medical tests are essential to properly diagnose patients with pseudoseizure, a disorder most common in those who have had a previously existing seizure disorder (Schofield and Duane 1987; Trimble 1983). Because advances in telemetry enable technicians to simultaneously videotape behavioral signs and monitor the electroencephalogram (EEG) in mobile patients, doctors can now fairly (but not absolutely) reliably verify whether the seizure-like behavior is connected with seizure activity in the brain. Unfortunately, however, the patient with a previously documented seizure disorder may have a telemetrically diagnosed pseudoseizure (i.e., an attack that does not change the EEG demonstrably). In such cases, he or she often is branded a "fake" and/or prematurely advised by frustrated house staff that he or she does not have a seizure disorder. Similarly, if the doctor identifies conversion-type symptoms, he or she can overlook organic brain dysfunction (Mersky and Buhrich 1975). In this situation, the psychiatrist can synthesize seemingly incompatible clinical information and help the primary-care physicians maintain their essential role as medical caregivers for patients who display disturbing psychiatric symptomatology.

Treatment

Consultation-liaison psychiatrists manage acute and chronic psychiatric disorders in patients hospitalized for medical conditions, behavioral disturbances in the management of medical/surgical patients, drug withdrawal, nonadherence to medical regimens, and a wide variety of chronic inpatient and outpatient problems, including overeating, smoking, psychophysiological disorders, suicidal and homicidal behavior, etc. Consultation-liaison psychiatrists are experts in the organic psychiatric treatments for psychiatric manifestations of medical illnesses and/or treatments. They advise staff and medical professionals on how to use psychotropic medications to manage acute organic brain disorders, antianxiety agents to facilitate substance withdrawal, lithium to stabilize a range of conditions, and antipsychotic or antidepressant medications to treat mental-status changes secondary to steroid treatment. The consultation-liaison psychiatrist's skills also contribute to successfully managing medical conditions such as renal or hepatic failure and the concomitant use of interacting pharmacological agents. Finally, consultation-liaison psychiatrists also prescribe and often provide crisis intervention, family therapy, behavioral therapy, biofeedback, relaxation therapy, and individual brief psychotherapy.

Unfortunately, health-care provision is changing in ways that may cripple effective consultation-liaison psychiatric practice and eventually lead to inadequate, even dangerous, provision of medical care. Today, many hospital administrators believe that nonmedical mental health workers can provide the patient with psychological services while the medical/surgical practitioners treat him or her medically. However, these administrators fail to understand that patients are best cared for when they benefit from the psychiatrist's capacity to provide both sorts of expertise in diagnosis and treatment. These administrators do not see that delegating the consultation-liaison psychiatrist's function to nonphysicians is unsafe, inefficient, and arguably illegal.

Funding of Modern Medicine and Consultation-Liaison Psychiatry: Cost-Effectiveness

Given current economic and political conditions, the issue of hospital reimbursement is increasingly important. In the past 20 years, reimbursement patterns for consultation-liaison psychiatry have been scaled back considerably, which has meant that many programs have shrunk or closed and that many psychiatrists have significantly shifted from liaison activities to consultation activities. Both movements have occurred, in part, because the government has decreased its support for psychiatric treatment and, in part, because third-party payers have elected to support direct medical care only. Nationwide, Fenton and Guggenheim (1981) found, for example, that consultations nationwide were only reimbursed at about 30% of billed charges. Recently, several medical-care reimbursers, most prominently Medicare and some private insurers, have moved from paying for services rendered to paying for the average expected "appropriate and efficient" treatment for a particular medical illness. Under some of these systems, hospitals and physicians are reimbursed for a specified number of "weighted work units" for a particular diagnosis-related group (DRG). Obviously, such fixed payment schemes reward medical-care systems that reduce hospital stays below the average. In addition, hospitals and physicians that provide "less efficient" care (i.e., patients linger and are tested more often) are punished because they have to absorb the increased cost of that treatment.

Although psychiatric comorbidities increase the time that a medically ill patient spends in the hospital, those longer stays need not cost the hospital money. For example, a patient hospitalized for a stroke receives a fixed number of weighted work units (worth, let's say, $60 per weighted work unit) for a hospital stay. However, if the patient also carries a diagnosis of alcohol dependence, or is over 70 years old, that DRG will be worth more weighted work units because the reimbursement plan allows older patients undergoing withdrawal from alcohol a longer stay in the hospital. Thus, the modern hospital cannot manage finances effectively unless it recognizes the reimbursable comorbidities. This aspect of financial management underscores how important it is that someone recognize, diagnose, and document psychiatric illness in medical patients. To the extent that psychiatric consultation identifies psychiatric illnesses that may be documented as a comorbidity, consultations more than pay for themselves. For example, in the Veterans Administration medical centers, the 10 most commonly diagnosed psychiatric conditions in the general medical hospital add between 70% and 170% greater financial value to the hospital for the 10 most common medical diagnoses. With the help of the consultation-liaison psychiatrist, the hospital can accrue greater financial rewards by identifying the most valuable DRGs.

In the private sector, paying for consultation-liaison services presents a difficult issue because the medical team, and not the patient, usually call in the consultation. Some patients actually refuse to pay for the consultation. If the patient is unwilling to pay, the hospital may fund the service because it helps ensure that the hospital functions efficiently and safely. Given that psychiatric consultation plays an integral role in teaching, some academic institutions consider the cost of consultations a part of the hospital overhead. For them, the psychiatric consultant fee is included as part of the professional fees involved in hospitalization. In some circumstances, the consultant may not view the liaison service as fee generating per se, but rather as a source of private paying referrals from the primary-care physician. In any case, complex insurance reimbursement procedures present a formidable obstacle to the independent practitioner. Practitioners are most often discouraged because private insurers reimburse at specified (or negotiated, as in the case of preferred providers) physician rates for consultants summoned by the primary medical team.

Cost Savings Resulting From Psychiatric Consultation

Psychiatric morbidities have been estimated to exist in 30% to 50% of all medical and surgical inpatients (Lipowski 1967). These comorbidities have meant that hospitals keep these patients for longer stays, that they test or surgically operate on them more often, and that they often require posthospital long-term–care facilities for such treatments (Fulop et al. 1987). However, just as psychotherapy has been shown to reduce the cost of medical treatment, recent research demonstrates that consultation-liaison psychiatry is effective in cutting the costs of hospitalization (Huyse 1989; Mumford et al. 1984; Schlesinger et al. 1983). In the mid-1930s, the Billings group first demonstrated that consultation-liaison psychiatric input could save money for hospitals (Billings et al. 1937). Within a year of implementing consultation-liaison consultants, patients needing psychiatric treatment were referred to psychiatrists on average 3 days earlier than they had previously been referred. Even more importantly, the patients referred for psychiatric treatment needed an average of 14% less time in the hospital.   •

More recently, Levitan and Kornfeld (1981) found that psychiatric screening and intervention on an orthopedic ward resulted in a significantly shortened hospitalization and reduced the cost of caring for patients with fractured hips. This study also supports Strain's suggestion that psychiatric services are more cost-effective when the screening method identifies medical patients who need psychiatrical consultation (Strain et al., in press). In Britain, Maguire et al. (1982) demonstrated that medical costs could be cut if women undergoing mastectomy were counseled. In a review of 34 controlled studies, Mumford et al. (1982) concluded that psychological intervention in postcardiotomy patients significantly decreased postoperative morbidity and length of hospital stay. In an elegant crossover study, Smith et al. (1986) found that health-care charges incurred by patients with somatization disorder (as compared to randomized control subjects) decreased by more than 50% after psychiatrists consulted and advised on how to manage these patients' treatment (Smith et al. 1986). As this evidence suggests, psychiatric consultation not only minimizes what the patient suffers but also saves money, shortens the length of stay, and minimizes morbidities (such as pneumonia, thrombosis, patient injuries) that accompany the development of persistent organic brain syndromes. In fact, as Lyons et al. (1986) have demonstrated, the earlier the patient is consulted on during his or her hospitalization, the less time the patient spends in the hospital. Finally, if we prevent such morbidities, we may also return the patient to a higher level of functioning, a value and a savings that the current structure of medical reimbursement does not acknowledge.

However, psychiatric consultation may reduce the costs of inpatient medical care in other ways as well. Many studies have attempted to estimate how many patients are admitted for extensive workup of medical problems that have, as their basis, psychiatric disorder (Smith et al. 1986). Although hospitals can make profits on tests and procedures, current prepaid systems (such as DRG-based systems) reward simplified workups. For example, expensive evaluations of cardiac complaints reveal many patients with an irritable esophagus, depression or psychosis with somatization, Briquet's syndrome, or hyperventilation or symptoms of panic disorder. Hospitals often do extensive neurological workups for pseudoseizure, pseudodementia, somatization, and headache, and the common gastrointestinal workups for irritable bowel syndrome or bowel syndromes secondary to affective disorder, which are very expensive. In other cases, the hospital may have to set up extensive and expensive medical evaluations for patients who suffer from affective disorder and who do not adhere to medical regimens. In order to avoid unnecessary medical expense, the hospital might instead rely on relatively inexpensive psychiatric consultations to investigate the psychogenic basis for symptoms and perhaps to prevent costly, uncomfortable, inconvenient, and even possibly dangerous workups (Loewenstein and Black 1983).

The psychiatric consultant further contributes to efficient hospital care by helping manage disruptive patients. Patients with severe depressive reactions, organic brain dysfunction, or anxiety are often unable to consent to tests and procedures. However, despite the patients' inability, ethics and laws generally constrain the hospital from discharging these patients; thus, the hospital is forced to absorb the cost of prolonged inpatient care. With psychiatric treatment the patient can often be encouraged to cooperate with inpatient care, aftercare, and placement. The psychiatrist may also medicate a patient to minimize psychotic thinking or frightening fantasies about illness. The psychiatrist may even work directly with family members to help a scared and confused patient to cooperate with the medical physicians. While many of the products of consultation-liaison psychiatry are difficult to quantify (Houpt 1987), these and other financial benefits can be measured, and all help the hospital care well and efficiently for the patients.

Stress on Inpatient Wards and the Psychiatric Consultant

The inpatient medical/surgical ward is naturally a stressful environment. Adding to that inherent stress, the new methods of funding hospital care and the current nursing shortage mean that both public and private institutions tend to be short of staff. As a result, today's hospital is an increasingly inhospitable place in which either to work or to be sick. While these trends encourage everyone to seek alternatives to inpatient hospitalization and, at least theoretically, to reduce the cost of medical care, the same trends have had a problematic effect on those who need hospitalization or who work in hospitals. For example, a short-handed staff may lose the emotional or physical flexibility to cope with patients who are not quiet, passive, and amenable to regimentation (the "ideal patient" mode). For the overworked staff, the patient becomes a malfunctioning machine into which to plug tubes and on which to change dressings.

Under these conditions, nurses are less able to explore and assess their patients' difficulties with being ill; they are also less likely to work with the patients to provide rehabilitation. Staff may mute a patient's anxieties about illnesses, treatments, and the future, with tranquilizers rather than by directly addressing and resolving these fears and needs. In addition, the patient who is not quiet, cooperative, and regimented because he or she is in a state of psychological chaos ends up spreading chaos through the ward. If patients disrupt the ward with loud, vulgar, or threatening vocalizations, make demands, act out, and/or refuse to be treated, they negatively affect the other patients' care and drain the staff of its emotional and physical reserve. In such a setting, and under these circumstances, the psychiatric consultant limits the degree to which these patients disrupt other patients and staff by attending to their emotional chaos.

Medicolegal Issues

As we have discussed, new developments in case law and skyrocketing malpractice claims have sensitized hospital administrators and medical practitioners to medicolegal liability. As part of this broader problem, malpractice claims frequently arise from mismanagement of psychiatric disturbances (such as suicidal attempts) on medical wards. We summarize below the major medicolegal issues likely to confront the consultation psychiatrist and suggest how the consultant can cope with these complex issues.

Danger to Self.   The usual risks inherent in psychiatric practice apply in the medical setting. The most common of these risks is that the patient is not adequately protected. Suicidal patients must be assessed, documented, treated, and reasonably restrained from harming themselves. Their environment must be protective—often a difficult task in the medical setting where the architecture is open, the opportunities to do harm to oneself are everywhere, and the staff is psychiatrically unsophisticated. One must always assume that the patient in a medical ward has a right to be protected as in a psychiatric hospital. A locked ward may help certain patients, depending on their condition. One-to-one, 24-hour supervision for a patient who is diagnosed as a significant suicidal risk is essential. Because it is easier to escape from a medical ward than a locked psychiatric hospital, the medical setting may necessitate closer patient supervision than in the psychiatric environment.

To put this problem in perspective, "failure to restrain" accounts for by far the greatest number of malpractice lawsuits against psychiatrists. Between 1985 and 1987, failure to restrain from causing harm to self or others accounted for 87% of all claims paid out by the Veterans Administration for alleged psychiatric malpractice (Beck 1988). In marked contrast, virtually none of these payments were made for adverse drug reactions (such as tardive dyskinesia, sudden death, etc.). The legal message is clear: providing a safe environment is the sine qua non of proper treatment.

The medical staff may find it difficult to recognize that the medical problems of psychiatric patients need to be supervised more intensively if those patients have delusions and hallucinate. If depressed, the diabetic patient may, for example, be uninterested in carefully managing blood sugar. Optimal medical treatment requires that both medical and psychiatric factors be taken into consideration.

Staff and medical practitioners have to carefully assess and manage acutely and chronically cognitively impaired patients who may be unpredictably suicidal, combative, or simply confused. Although often calm and predictable while on their familiar "home" ward, these patients may become increasingly scared and confused when transported away from their familiar surroundings—to obtain an X-ray, for example. At such times, the consultant weighs the legal duty to provide a safe environment for these patients against respect for their rights to move about and to refuse psychoactive substances. Even after their medical problems have been resolved, such patients often must be transferred to the psychiatric hospital, where they can get the continued surveillance they need to protect themselves.

Generally, as most psychiatrists know, the most difficult patient to manage is the agitated psychotic, manic, or schizophrenic patient. Medical teams, including "sitters," need to be instructed in how to predict and manage these patients when they are agitated (see Chapter 9). When patients of this type are on the ward, a nursing shift may have to locate several strong (preferably experienced) nurses or nursing assistants who can be called if needed. In these cases, staff, medical personnel, and the consultant must make a measured effort to assure that the identified patient, fellow hospitalized patients, and staff are safe.

In addition to the problem of environment, treating these patients presents legal pitfalls for the psychiatric consultant. Numerous malpractice suits arise from the patients who have not been restrained, who have been improperly restrained, who have been secluded, or who have been "chemically restrained." If you are unsure about a recommendation or treatment, obtain a second psychiatric—or legal—opinion. The consultant may face further difficulties when planning to discharge patients who are prone to harm themselves. After assessing the risk of danger, the consultation-liaison psychiatrist may need to set up a plan that includes transferring the patient to a psychiatric hospital or ward with or without commitment certification.

Danger to Others. Responsibility for protection also extends to the situations in which a patient's unpredictable violence endangers roommates or visitors. In the medical setting the staff is often not trained either to identify or to control such behaviors; thus, they may need help from the psychiatric consultant to adequately fulfill that responsibility. Threats to hurt others, whether they be staff or persons outside the hospital, need to be taken seriously. Like the psychiatric environment, the medical environment imposes the duty to warn potential victims of violence. Today, the problem of "duty to warn" is complicated by patients with acquired immunodeficiency syndrome (AIDS) who threaten to infect others. Indeed. some argue that AIDS-infected patients who refuse to reveal their illness to their sexual partners should be treated as seriously as homicidal patients and that the potential victims of these dangerous patients should be warned. (For further discussion of the management of potentially dangerous patients, see Chapter 9.)

Informed Consent for Medical Procedures. In the medical hospital, consultation-liaison psychiatrists are often called upon to assess whether a patient is capable of giving informed consent for medical and surgical procedures (Mahler and Perry 1988). Such assessments differ procedurally from determining whether a patient has the right to move freely or be discharged (i.e., being potentially harmful to self or potentially harmful to others, or having a grave disability). Patients who are certified to the general hospital because they have psychiatric disabilities still retain the right to accept or refuse treatment unless they have been adjudicated "incompetent" by a court.

Capacity to give informed consent requires that a patient is able to understand the nature of the illness, the nature of the proposed treatment alternatives, and the risks and benefits of various available treatments versus nontreatment. In most states, doctors are protected against a legal action if they provide *emergency* treatment for a patient who cannot give informed consent. However, in subacute or nonacute situations, a judge must approve treatment if the patient cannot provide consent. Psychiatrists who wish to treat such patients should, of course, document that the procedure is medically necessary and that the patient is incapable of providing informed consent.

Occasionally, substituted consent obtained from a next of kin adequately protects the doctor who recommends procedures with minimal morbidity and mortality. For example, a patient in his 70s was admitted for treatment of gangrene of the foot resulting from a foot ulcer that had healed poorly. The patient steadfastly refused treatment, stating that his leg was getting better. A quiet man who said little to anybody, the patient appeared to act appropriately in most other aspects of his hospitalization. He was able to feed himself, to watch television, and to ask for pain medications. He was always fully oriented to time, place, and person. The patient was aware that he was hospitalized for treatment of his leg. Nevertheless, he continued to say his leg was improving even when gangrene had progressed above the knee. Although his family was unwilling to force an operation on the patient, they (like the patient) wanted him to live. On this basis, judicial approval of treatment was sought. The patient was brought to court, where the judge could observe that the patient was unable to accurately assess the nature of his illness and therefore did not have the capacity to consent to or refuse treatment. The court appointed the hospital temporary conservator, and the amputation was performed. Following his operation, the patient became more talkative, and it was retrospectively apparent that the patient had been so indecisive because of a subtle organic brain syndrome (he later told us of his suspiciousness) and denial. The patient thanked us profusely and was sad that he had not been "forced" into the operation sooner so that more of his leg might have been saved.

In consent cases, courts will consider what kinds of medical treatments are available for the patient's condition. Courts are considerably less likely to approve a medical procedure if a patient protests when that procedure has dubious benefits or requires that the patient cooperate with the doctor and the staff. Consider the case of a woman in her 60s with a severe personality disorder complicated by chronic alcoholism and chronic obstructive pulmonary disease. She had a broken cervical vertebra compressing her phrenic nerves, but she refused surgical fixation. As part of the treatment, she would need 6 weeks of traction. The court reasoned (properly) that in those 6 weeks, she was so likely to sabotage her treatment that it was impractical to limit her civil rights for such a small chance of success.

Psychotropic Medication Side Effects. In the general hospital, a variety of medicolegal issues surround the use of psychotropic medication, the most prescribed medicines in the world (Balter 1973). Informed consent, proper administration, and the monitoring of side effects are critical areas of concern. Thus, for example, the psychiatrist should know that the possibility of legal action can increase when psychotropic medications are used in nonpsychiatric patients or for non-FDA approved uses such as administration of neuroleptics in patients who have organic brain syndrome or of lithium in patients who have mania secondary to steroid treatment. The psychiatrist must keep informed—and inform consulting services—of the evolving case law on the patient's rights to refuse such medications (Applebaum 1988). Even though the primary physician ultimately prescribes and monitors all medications, the psychiatric consultant is the expert who is required by the law and the Joint Commission on Accreditation of Hospitals (JCAH) to inform primary care givers about the effects of medication (JCAH 1988, p. 91). Currently, the law does not clearly determine whether or not the consultant or the consultee has final responsibility in any case where the consultant's recommendations have harmed the patient, especially where the psychiatrist has a legal duty to appropriately inform the consultee.

The question of responsibility becomes particularly complicated when a patient's medical condition or concomitant use of other medications complicates the dosage, side effects, or effectiveness of the psychotropic medicine. For example, a patient was placed on a neuroleptic medication that caused peripheral α-adrenergic blockade, who then required epinephrine for another condition. The patient became irreversibly hypotensive and died. Apparently, the stimulatory effects of the epinephrine combined with the α-adrenergic blockade of the neuroleptic to reduce peripheral resistance and reduce blood pressure. Given the complexity of this kind of medicolegal issue, the psychiatrist may need legal advice in difficult cases.

Electroconvulsive Therapy.   In the general hospital, ECT use, although relatively infrequent, carries with it the usual responsibilities of properly assessing the patient, properly administering and posttreatment following up, obtaining informed consent, and ensuring that the patient knows that he or she can refuse treatment. The patient's medical condition is particularly important when considering whether to use ECT. ECT has many advantages over antidepressant medications for medically ill patients because it has no cardiac conduction blocking properties or anticholinergic side effects and because its onset is rapid. ECT is dangerous or problematic for some patients. Mass brain lesions are an absolute contraindication to the use of ECT. Its use will be complicated by concurrent cognitive impairment or underlying seizure disorder. Given the negative publicity related to ECT treatment, the doctor who recommends its use should be prepared to document the specific rationale for choosing it over the more conservative (and often more dangerous) medication treatments.

Confidentiality.   In previous chapters, we have already discussed issues of confidentiality in several contexts. As all doctors know, the law, statute, and tradition protect a patient's right to assume that what he or she communicates is private. However, this right is counterbalanced by the doctor's need to share information that will ensure that the patient gets the best care within the hospital and with other facilities when the patient is transferred (Kimball 1979). Consequently, no consultant can guarantee that a patient will get total confidentiality simply because that patient entered into a consultation relationship. As we discussed in Chapter 6, the consultant works with the patient to determine what—if any—information the patient prefers to have kept out of the medical record. However, the patient has the right to expect that hospital records will be kept confidential from visitors and even family members, except, perhaps, in the case of medical emergency. Whenever a doctor has to decide what "right" to trample on, he or she must first determine what will ensure that the patient is safe. Thus, as noted above, the psychiatrist's duty to warn potential victims that a patient is dangerous outweighs his or her duty of confidentiality.

Service Standards

Quality assurance, risk management, and utilization review are perhaps the three most important and most unpopular concepts in medical administration and practice today. Many doctors no longer take pleasure in their medical practice because they must divert too much time and energy away from the patient care to address these issues. Like other medical services, psychiatric services have been required by federal regulation (United States Code 1982, 1983) and by the JCAH (1988) to actively involve themselves in assessing the *quality* and *appropriateness* of treatment.

However, the factors involved in "quality" care are broad and often difficult to quantify. Central to the idea of quality is whether care is effective and efficient within the customary standard of practice in the community. In order to assess quality, each service must first have a set of specific guidelines for practice (in addition to the hospital bylaws that guide all physician practice). These guidelines must be based on accepted standards of practice and should probably meet the standards explicitly recommended in the JCAH guidelines. Whether a practice is acceptable and/or up-to-date depends on standards of educational background, continuing education, and caseload.

However, the service must do more than assess practice; each program must also demonstrate that when indicated, it actively implements steps to rectify deficiencies. That is, services need to assess the quality of service policies and procedures specific to themselves: how they select and train employees, how they stand on continuing education and certification, how they evaluate employee performance, and how they assess the effectiveness of their continuous monitoring techniques. Quality assurance standards require all medical services—including consultation-liaison—to assure that their practitioners are well versed in medical practice. An accepted standard for practice in consultation psychiatry is supported by the increasing subspecialization of consultation-liaison psychiatry, the establishment of consultation-liaison societies, and the promulgation of knowledge bases for training in consultation-liaison psychiatry.

The JCAH mandates a systematized employee performance evaluation that uses explicit, written monitors to assess quality, appropriateness, and efficiency of care, although monitors may be continuous, use targeted investigations, or be incident-specific (Table 12-1). A program must assess all medical treatment provided by all medical practitioners on an ongoing basis. Some (or parts of some) of these assessments may be performed by nonprofessionals—for example, timeliness, incident tracking, and the presence of diagnoses. However, professionals need to control other aspects of performance evaluations such as the performance chart or consultation report reviews. Individuals should not be designated as "in charge of" quality assurance; instead, all professionals on the service should be involved in these evaluations.

Continuous monitors track the level of care provided. Such monitors can help identify trends in practice such as when diagnostic categories change, or whether incidents of organic mental syndromes, drug reactions, or misuse of medication increase. The monitors may either be "process" or "outcome" oriented. The process audit evaluates what the psychiatrist performs for the patients. For example, does the consultant obtain the proper information or perform the necessary evaluations? However, this type of audit does not determine whether the psychiatrist reaches the desired goals of diagnosis and treatment. Compared to the process audits, outcome care audits are more difficult and time consuming because they are specific for particular patient popu-

Table 12-1. Quality assurance outline for medical-care personnel

Continuous monitors

Timeliness of the consultation

Adequacy of the report
   a. Are essential elements of history obtained?
   b. Is mental status examination present?
   c. Are medications reviewed?

Legibility of the consultation report

Do the diagnoses follow from the documented data?

Are the recommendations of the consultant appropriately followed by the medical team?

Do the treatment recommendations follow from the diagnosis?

Focused review audit

Assess therapeutic misadventures

   a. Use of psychotropic medications contraindicated by the patient's condition or use of other medications
   b. Misuse of restraints
   c. Inadequate provision of protection for delirious or suicidal patients
   d. Appropriateness of commitment procedures

Incident tracking

Suicidal attempts, gestures, and/or threats

Against-medical-advice discharges

Note. Based on Joint Commission on Accreditation of Hospitals 1988.

lations and diagnoses and need to be performed by professionals. For example, it is difficult to set up and evaluate the outcome of methylphenidate use in medically ill depressed patients in part because such an evaluation may require a large patient cohort. On the other hand, it is relatively easy to determine whether or not the consultee followed the consultant's recommendations about how to manage a patient's medication. Despite these costs, outcome case audits do allow a service to measure how well it achieves its desired goals.

Again, focused review audits may be either process or outcome specific. The JCAH has encouraged focused reviews because they are ideally limited to identifying the extent, causes of, and possible solutions to a previously noted clinical problem. These studies may be retrospective, concurrent, or prospective in nature. Consultation-liaison services will find that investigations of consultee concordance with psychiatric recommendations are a particularly important type of review (Wise et al. 1987). Services may also find incident reporting and other risk-management techniques (e.g., identifying trends in incidents such as suicide attempts) useful to determine what problems may not be identified by the continuous review. In incident-oriented auditing, the service focuses on adverse events and evaluates, in depth, the processes that contributed to those adverse events. Through such investigations, the consultation-liaison service can identify a specific plan for focused audits in order to assess whether or not it has a larger problem. In order to use audits most effectively, clinical services should work with a quality assurance specialist who is experienced in developing and implementing quality assurance programs.

In several jurisdictions, quality assurance proceedings are protected from discovery in legal proceedings. The courts have consistently upheld that the hospital has the right to hold such investigations confidential and have refused to allow the proceedings to be used as evidence against the hospital or the practitioner. The courts recognize that the quality assurance self-examination procedures must be conducted without fear of self-incrimination in order to improve the quality of the patient care delivered. Nevertheless, certain quality assurance–related activities may not be protected from discovery. For example, the courts may not protect practice policies, licensure status, and administrative files including personnel actions. Those who develop policies and enter data into personnel files should be aware of how the law applies in this area. For example, a psychiatric service thought it should perform a new extensive standardized examination for every patient with suicidal ideation. In order to pressure the staff to perform the extensive evaluation, the program director published a policy mandating the evaluation, which was much more extensive than was usually necessary under the circumstances. However, because the policy seemed unnecessary, many of the service's psychiatrists did not comply with it. In this case, publishing a policy that lacked merit and was thus unlikely to be followed was legally dangerous. If a psychiatrist does not give the full examination required by the policy to a patient who then attempted suicide, a strong case could be made that the examining physician had not followed the hospital's established policy and should therefore be held liable if the patient is harmed. Because, in this example, the hospital policy mandated a much more comprehensive examination than was community standard, the hospital actually expanded its liability.

CONCLUSIONS

Today, the psychiatric consultant plays an increasingly important role in a medical-care system evolving toward greater and greater subspecialization. In this world of specialists, the consultant can synthesize and interpret often disparate somatic and psychological information, thus playing a role that nonmedical mental health workers cannot play. As more and more legal actions are brought against hospitals that fail to provide proper psychiatric evaluation and treatment, the consultation-liaison psychiatrist becomes more and more integrated in the medical setting. Finally, as a number of studies document, the consultation-liaison psychiatrist is a cost-effective member of the medical team because he or she manages the psychiatric interventions that decrease the length of time many patients spend in the hospital. Thus, despite changes in the medical-care system, the practice of consultation-liaison psychiatry will continue to be profoundly important in the medical setting and to medically-ill patients.

REFERENCES

Applebaum PS: The right to refuse treatment with antipsychotic medications: retrospect and prospect. Am J Psychiatry 145:413–419, 1988
Balter MB: An analysis of psychotherapeutic drug consumption in the United States, in Proceedings of the Anglo-American Conference on Drug Abuse: Etiology of Drug Abuse, Vol 1. Edited by Bowen RA. London, Royal Society of Medicine, 1973, pp 58–65

Beck CE: Psychiatric malpractice claims in the VA. VA Practitioner 5:45–53, 1988

Billings EG, McNary SW, Rees MH: Financial importance of general hospital psychiatry to hospital administrator. Hospitals 11: 40–44, 1937

Fenton BJ, Guggenheim FG: Consultation-liaison psychiatry and funding: why can't Alice find wonderland? Gen Hosp Psychiatry 3:255–260, 1981

Fulop G, Strain JJ, Vita J, et al: Impact of psychiatric comorbidity on length of hospital stay for medical/surgical patients: a preliminary report. Am J Psychiatry 144:878–882, 1987

Houpt JL: Products of consultation-liaison psychiatry. Gen Hosp Psychiatry 9:350–353, 1987

Huyse FJ: Systematic Interventions in Consultation/Liaison Psychiatry. Amsterdam, Free University Press, 1989

Joint Commission on Accreditation of Hospitals: Accreditation Manual for Hospitals. Chicago, IL, Joint Commission on Accreditation of Hospitals, 1988

Kimball CP: The issue of confidentiality in the consultation-liaison process, in The Teaching of Psychosomatic Medicine and Consultation Psychiatry. Edited by Kimball CP, Krakowski AJ. Basel, S Karger, 1979, pp 82–89

Larson DB, Kessler LC, Burns BJ, et al: A research development workshop to stimulate outcome research in consultation-liaison psychiatry. Hosp Community Psychiatry 38:1106–1109, 1987

Levitan SJ, Kornfeld DS: Clinical and cost benefits of liaison psychiatry. Am J Psychiatry 138:790–793, 1981

Lipowski ZJ: Review of consultation psychiatry and psychosomatic medicine. II. Clinical aspects. Psychosom Med 29:201–224, 1967

Loewenstein RJ, Black HR: Recognition, evaluation and differential diagnosis of psychiatric and somatic conditions, in Psychiatry in the Practice of Medicine. Edited by Leigh H. Menlo Park, CA, Addison-Wesley, 1983, pp 57–81

Lyons JS, Hammer JS, Strain JJ, et al: The timing of psychiatric consultation in the general hospital and length of hospital stay. Gen Hosp Psychiatry 8:159–162, 1986

Maguire P, Pentol A, Allen D, et al: Cost of counseling women who undergo mastectomy. Br Med J 284:1933–1935, 1982

Mahler J, Perry S: Assessing competency in the physically ill: guidelines for psychiatric consultants. Hosp Community Psychiatry 39:856–861, 1988

Mersky H, Buhrich NA: Hysteria and organic brain disease. Br J Med Psychol 48:359–366, 1975

Mumford E, Schlesinger HJ, Glass GV: The effects of psychological intervention on recovery from surgery and heart attacks: an analysis of the literature. Am J Public Health 72:141–151, 1982

Mumford E, Schlesinger HJ, Glass GV, et al: A new look at evidence about reduced cost of medical utilization following mental health treatment. Am J Psychiatry 141:1145–1158, 1984

Schlesinger HJ, Mumford E, Glass GV, et al: Mental health treatment and medical care utilization in a fee-for-service system: outpatient mental health treatment following the onset of a chronic disease. Am J Public Health 73:422–429, 1983

Schofield A, Duane MMA: Neurologic referrals to a psychiatric consultation-liaison service. Gen Hosp Psychiatry 9:280–286, 1987

Smith RG, Monson RA, Ray DC: Psychiatric consultation in somatization disorder. N Engl J Med 314:1407–1413, 1986

Strain JJ, Fulop G, Hammer JS, et al: Psychosocial interventions and the cost of medical treatment, in The Development of Competent and Humane Physicians. Edited by Hendrie HC. Bloomington, IN, Indiana University Press (in press)

Trimble M: Pseudoseizures. Br J Hosp Med 29:326–333, 1983

United States Code, 42, para 1320c, 1982 (peer review of the utilization and quality of health care services); par 1320c-1, 1982 (utilization and quality control peer review organization defined)

United States Code, 42, par 1320c-1, suppl I, 1983

Wise TN, Mann LS, Silverstein R, et al: Consultation-liaison outcome evaluation system (CLOES): resident or private attending physicians' concordance with consultant's recommendations. Compr Psychiatry 28:430–436, 1987

Index

Administrative issues, 109, 116–118
Administrators, 25
AIDS, 159, 215
American Academy of Pediatrics, 195
American Board of Internal Medicine, 195
American Medical Association, 195
Association for Academic Psychiatry, 197

Behavior management, 156–164
Benefits of consultation-liaison psychiatry, 206–223

Call coverage, 46–48
Calling mechanisms, 45–48
Chart. *See* Patient's chart
Clergy members, 32–33, 83–84, 165
Clerks, 25–26
Commitment, 119–120, 161
Computer-assisted recordkeeping, 51–52, 128, 144–147
Confidentiality, 89–92, 114, 218–219
Conflicting allegiances, 4, 92–93
Conflicts among staff, 76–78
Consent, 88–89, 161–162, 178, 215–217
Consultant-consultee relationship
    attitude of consultant, 34–35
    attitude of consultee, 34
    consultee practice patterns, 35–36
    education role of consultant, 193–196
    establishing, 33–37
    familiarity with consultee specialty, 36–37
    and written consultation, 130, 179–180
Contacting the referring service
    contracting for consultation, 67–70
    importance of, 55
    information sought, 58–67
    timing, 56–57
    whom to contact, 57–58
Contracting for consultation, 67–70, 92–93
Cost-effectiveness, 208–212

Dangerousness, 162–164, 213–215
Diagnosis, 99, 135–136
Differential diagnosis, 154–155
Discharge against medical advice, 160–161, 165–166
Discharge planning, 188–189
Documentation. *See* Writing up the consultation
Drop box system, 43
Durable power of attorney for health care, 162
Duty to warn, 163–164, 215

Education role of consultation-liaison psychiatrist
    medical students, 202–203
    nonpsychiatric physicians, 179–180, 193–196
    residents, 196–202
    teaching, 37–38
Electroconvulsive therapy (ECT), 184, 218
Emergency situations, 48, 64–65, 162, 216
Ending consultation, 190–191
Environment, 103–104, 121, 212–213
Ethnic and language differences, 78, 111

Families
    and complexities of multiple caregivers, 77
    and confidentiality, 114
    and consent, 162
    and discharge, 165–166
    information from, 112–114, 155–156
    as sitters, 120–121
Follow-up
    assessing the need for, 177–182
    delineation of responsibility, 170–171
    goals for, 182–185
    implementation, 185–188
Folstein-McHugh Mini-Mental State Exam, 153
Formulations, 135–136
Fragmentation of care, 72–76
Friends of patient
    and confidentiality, 114
    information from, 112–114
    See also Visitors
Funding, 208–210

Guardianship, 115, 119

Halstead-Reitan neuropsychological test, 153
Historical perspective on consultation-liaison psychiatry, 10–15, 20–22
House staff, 33

Information card, 42–44
Information gathering
    from caller requesting consultation, 49–51
    from families and friends, 112–114, 155–156
    before leaving the medical unit, 109, 110–116
    from other sources, 115–116
    past medical records, 114–115
    patient's chart, 78–83, 110
    preliminary information, 58–67
    from staff, 110–112
    staff relationships, 76–78
    from visitors, 83–84, 94
    who is taking care of patient, 72–76
Informing the patient, 67–69
Institutional familiarity, 4–5, 37
Institutional stress, 212–213
Insurance, 39, 48, 99, 116, 209–210
Intake procedures
    call coverage, 46–48
    calling mechanisms, 45–48
    information card, 42–44
    information to request, 49–51
    prearrangements, 42
    recording and conveying information, 51–52
    who may initiate contact, 44–45
Interview, 93–101

Joint Commission on Accreditation of Hospitals (JCAH), 44, 156, 217, 219, 220, 222

Laboratory tests, 82, 154
Legal issues, 109, 115–118, 140, 213–219
Liaison, 4–5, 149–152
Limited consultation, 140

Medical consultants, 153–154
Medical records, 114–115
    See also Patient's chart

Medical students, 75–76, 202–203
Mental Health and Developmental Disabilities Confidentiality
    Act, 89
Mental status examination, 59, 61–62, 100–101, 133–135
Minnesota Multiphasic Personality Inventory (MMPI), 153

Neurological consultants, 29, 153
Nonmedical consultations, 155–156
Nursing staff, 30–31, 73–74

Outpatient therapists, 67
Overview, 5–10

Paging systems, 46–47
Patients
   attitude, 2–3, 87–88
   communicating first impressions, 104–106
   consent, 88–89, 161–162, 178, 215–217
   environment, 103–104, 121, 212–213
   informing, 67–69
   interview, 93–101
   physical examination, 102–103
   refusal, 97–98, 178, 191
   safety, 156–157, 213–215
Patient's chart, 78–83, 110, 124
Physical examination, 102–103
Physical restraints, 119, 157–159
Precipitants for consultation, 63–64
Privilege. See Confidentiality
Psychiatric history, 132–133
Psychiatrists as consultants, 1–5, 39–40
Psychological testing, 153
Psychologists, 28–30
Psychopharmacology, 150–151, 167–169, 183–184, 195, 217–218
Psychosomatic medicine, 5–6, 11, 13–15, 20–22
Psychotherapeutic treatment, 167

Quality assurance standards, 219–223

Recommendations
   behavior management, 156–164
   further diagnostic workup, 152–156
   liaison, 149–152

treatment, 164–171
types, 152–171
urgent, 118–121
in written consultation, 137–139
Referral, 169–170
Reorganizing an existing service, 38–39
Residents, 196–202

Safety, 156–157, 214
Secretaries, 25–26
Setting up a consultation service
establishing consultant-consultee relationship, 33–37
institutional familiarity, 37
meeting the staff, 24–33
in a new setting, 23–24
professional identity, 39–40
reorganizing an existing service, 38–39
teaching, 37–38
Side effects of psychotropic medication, 155, 167–168, 217–218
Sitters, 65, 116, 120–121, 156–157, 173–175, 215
Social intervention, 164–166
Social workers, 26–28, 117, 164–165
Specialized service staff, 31–32
Staff
information from, 110–112
meeting, 24–33
relationships, 76–78
sharing impressions with, 122–124
Stress, 212–213
Suicidal precautions, 44, 156–157, 173–175, 214

Tarasoff warnings, 163–164, 215
Teaching, 29, 37–38
See also Education role of consultation-liaison psychiatrist
Therapeutic alliances, 2
Therapeutic interventions, 3
Transference, 102, 181
Transfers, 169–170
Treatment recommendations
psychiatric follow-up, 170–171
psychopharmacology, 167–168
psychotherapy, 167
referral and transfer, 169–170

    social intervention, 164–166
Trends, 5, 205–223
Triage, 47–48

Urgency, 48, 56, 64–65, 118–121

Visitors
    and confidentiality, 83–84, 94
    information from, 83–84, 94
    monitoring, 159–160

Wechsler Adult Intelligence Scale—Revised (WAIS-R), 153
Who may initiate contact, 44–45
Writing up the consultation
    computer-assisted data base supplement, 51–52, 128, 144–147
    elements, 128–129
    format, 127–128
    formulations, 135–136
    legal implications, 140
    limited consultation, 140
    outline, 143